Pilates:
Using Small Props for Big Results

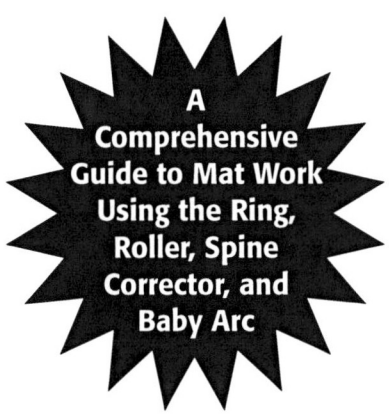

A Comprehensive Guide to Mat Work Using the Ring, Roller, Spine Corrector, and Baby Arc

Christine Romani-Ruby, MPT, ATC

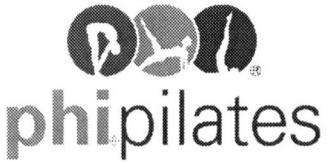

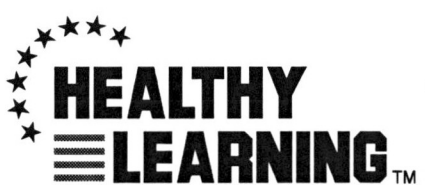

©2009 Healthy Learning. All rights reserved. Printed in the United States.

No part of this book may be reproduced, stored in a retrieval system, or transmitted, in any form or by any means, electronic, mechanical, photocopying, recording, or otherwise, without the prior permission of Healthy Learning. Throughout this book, the masculine shall be deemed to include the feminine and vice versa.

ISBN: 978-1-60679-061-8
Library of Congress Control Number: 2009923839

Book layout: Bean Creek Studio
Cover design: Bean Creek Studio
Front and back cover photos: David Savarino
Text photos: David Savarino

Healthy Learning
P.O. Box 1828
Monterey, CA 93942
www.healthylearning.com

Dedication

This book is dedicated to Joseph and Clara Pilates.
Thank you for your innovative method.

Acknowledgments

Special thanks to Lauren Nahas, MPT, Pilates instructor, dancer, and physical therapist, who gracefully modeled all of the exercises for the photos in this book.

Special thanks to two companies for listening to and fulfilling the requests and needs of their customers:

- Airex® for the YogaPilates 190 mat used in the photos
- Balanced Body® for the Clara Step Barrel® and baby arc used in the photos

Contents

Dedication 3

Acknowledgments 4

Preface 8

Chapter 1: Pilates Principles 9
    The Guiding Principles of Pilates
    Pilates Principles for Breathing
    Review of Basic Pilates Mat Neutral Positions
    The Use of Props for Pilates Mat Work
    Choosing the Props

Chapter 2: The Foam Roller 19
    Articulating Bridge With One Roller
    Articulating Bridge With Two Rollers
    Leg Circles
    Roll-Up on Two Rollers
    Hundred With Two Rollers
    Ribcage Arms on Two Rollers
    Scissors
    Helicopter
    Mermaid
    Hip Abductor
    Eve's Lunge
    Knee Stretch (Abdominal Tuck) on Two Rollers
    Knee Stretch (Abdominal Tuck) on One Roller
    Modified Swimming on Two Rollers
    Push-Up With Hands on the Roller
    Cat on the Roller
    Push-Up With Knees on the Roller
    Reverse Plank on Two Rollers
    Frog

Chapter 3: The Pilates Ring 59
Hundred
Articulating Bridge
Cervical Nod
Roll-Up
Hip Adductor
Shoulder Stability
Shave the Head
Spine Stretch
Mermaid
Ribcage Arms
Pliés and Footwork
Squats
Hamstring Stretch
Long Back Stretch
Hip Extension/Frog

Chapter 4: The Spine Corrector 91
Arm Circles
Leg Circles
Scissors
Helicopter
Walking
Bicycle
Beats
Rolling In and Out
Stretch With Bar
Teaser
Swan
Hip Circles
Mermaid
Mermaid Legs
Shoulder Bridge
Swimming
Seated Twist
Roll-Up

Chapter 5: Small Barrel (Baby Arc) 129
- Arm Circles
- Leg Circles
- Scissors
- Walking
- Bicycle
- Beats
- Rolling In and Out

Appendix: Adding Props to Your Pilates Mat Work 145

About the Author 148

Preface

In 1945, Joseph Pilates published two books about his method that he called Contrology. In these books, he described his method as a way to cure and prevent physical ills, and he continuously referred to the "deplorable state of ignorance surrounding health and the lack of understanding of the cooperation of mind and body in the result of total well-being."* He appealed to Americans that it was their duty not only to attain health, but to maintain it. Joseph Pilates was genuinely interested in the good of mankind; his main desire was to empower people with the ability to take control of their own well-being. This strategy is now known as wellness. Wellness is defined as "concepts that embrace positive behaviors and promote a state of physical and mental balance and fitness."**

At times, wellness seems far out of reach due to disease, injury, or muscle imbalance from sport. Joseph Pilates' answer to this problem was his innovative use of tools to enhance movement. He created the tools from common items that he had available. For example, the first Pilates ring was made from a garbage can lid, the Cadillac was made from a hospital bed, and the pedi-pole was made from a hospital IV pole. He then used these tools to enhance and teach proper movement to his clients. Proper movement involved a connection of the movement to the mind, and Joseph professed that this connection was the pathway to happiness.

This book provides exercises to help people work much like Joseph Pilates. The exercises use small props to enhance and encourage proper movement, connecting the mind and the body. Creating muscle balance through proper movement patterns will make and keep anyone well, whether they are a high-level athlete or recovering from an injury.

---

*Pilates, J., & Miller, W. (2000). In Gallagher, S., Kryzanowska, R. (Eds.), *The complete writings of Joseph H. Pilates*. Philadelphia, PA: BainBridgeBooks.

**American Physical Therapy Association (1999). *Guide to Physical Therapist Practice* (Second Edition). Alexandria, VA: American Physical Therapy Association.

Pilates Principles

Contrology has been successfully passed down through the generations because of the clear vision and expert teachings of Joe Pilates. He created simple and easy-to-follow principles to guide teachers and students in the method of Contrology. These principles have been shared from teacher to teacher and now are showing promising effects on core strength and agility in case studies and research.

The Guiding Principles of Pilates

In his book, *Return to Life Through Contrology*, written in 1920, Joseph Pilates described the principles of his method of Contrology. These principles define the work as intended by its creator. Joe Pilates wrote that with patience and persistence, individuals could successfully derive all the benefits of Contrology in their own home. He said to "remember that you are teaching yourself—right!"* The following six principles are what he outlined as the key components for success in his program:

- *Concentration:* Joe Pilates said to "concentrate on the correct movements each time you exercise." He said the exercises needed to be correctly executed and mastered to the point of subconscious reaction.
- *Control:* Joe Pilates wrote, "Ideally our muscles should obey our will. Reasonably our will should not be dominated by the reflex actions of our muscles. Contrology starts with mind control over muscles."
- *Centering:* All movement comes from a stable center. Joseph called this center "the Powerhouse," and it included the rectangular area between the shoulders and the hips.
- *Flow:* Joe Pilates wrote, "Contrology was conceived to limber and stretch the muscles and ligaments so that your body will be as supple as that of a cat." The movements are performed gracefully, smoothly, and evenly.
- *Precision:* Joe Pilates wrote to study carefully: "Do not sacrifice knowledge to speed." The instructions had to be followed exactly, down to the very smallest detail.
- *Breath:* Joe Pilates stated that breathing is the first act of life—and the last. He wanted you to "squeeze every atom of air from your lungs until they are almost as free of air as is a vacuum." He insisted on a forced exhalation and a complete deep inhalation. Each movement was tied to the breath.

Pilates Principles for Breathing

Joseph Pilates had general principles that he used to teach his clients how to properly breathe during the exercises. He encouraged students to inhale when extending their

---

*All the quoted material in this section is from Pilates, J., & Miller, W. (2000). In Gallagher, S., Kryzanowska, R. (Eds.), *The complete writings of Joseph H. Pilates*. Philadelphia, PA: BainBridgeBooks.

spine or limbs, and to exhale when flexing their spine or limbs. He believed that inhalation would support and extend the spine, and the exhale would engage the deep abdominal muscles. His beliefs are now supported by research that provides evidence that the diaphragm supports the upper lumbar spine on inhalation and the transverse abdominus supports the lower lumbar spine on exhalation.* Both of these muscles have been identified as vital local muscles responsible for core stability to protect the spine from injury. They are both involuntary muscles, which is why the breath is used to facilitate their contraction during activities where the spine needs support.

The following guidelines are a successful way to facilitate Pilates-style breathing. A client may find it difficult to adopt any breathing style during exercise. Remember that these principles are a guide. They are not set rules. You may find that some of your clients will need to exhale in order to engage their abdominal muscles during the exertion part of the exercise, even if that phase of the exercise is placing the spine in extension. Sometimes a client may need to take several breaths to properly perform an exercise. In a group class setting, you may want to reverse the breathing in order to challenge some participants or help others properly perform an exercise. When working one-on-one with an individual, you should choose the breathing style that the client may need in that particular exercise. For example, if your client cannot maintain a neutral spine in a prone extension exercise, instruct the client to try exhaling as he extends to better support the torso.

In the teachings of Phi® Pilates, a full complete breath with inhalation through the nose and exhalation through the mouth is recommended for two reasons. First, inhalation through the nose filters and warms the air before the body uses it. Second, when exhaling through the mouth using a "ha" sound, the deep abdominal muscles engage and the neck and mouth remain relaxed. A full complete breath is functional and can be used by your clients in all daily activities.

Components of Pilates-Style Breathing

- The inhale and exhale are always equal in length.
- The breath is tied to the movement, and no holding of the breath is permitted. Avoid the valsalva effect.
- The ribcage expands to the sides and back on the inhale. This expansion encourages air flow to the lower lobes of the lungs. A useful cue here is to expand the ribcage from both sides.

---

*Hodges, P.W., Eriksson, M.E., Shirley, D., & Gandevia, S.C. (2005). Intra-abdominal pressure increases stiffness of lumbar spine. *Journal of Biomechanics, 38,* 1873-80.

Jenkins, J.R. (2003). The transversus adbominis and reconditioning the lower back. *Strength and Conditioning Journal, 25*(6), 60-66.

Jenkins, J.R. (2004). Addendum to the transversus adbominis and reconditioning the lower back. *Strength and Conditioning Journal, 26*(2), 78-79.

- On the exhale, the ribcage closes and the navel draws in toward the spine, engaging the deep abdominal muscles. A useful cue here is to draw the ribs toward the front pockets of the pants.

Joe Pilates describes two additional important concepts or principles in his book *Contrology,** and they are included here as they are useful in understanding and teaching the work for rehabilitation purposes.

Relaxation: Relaxation was described by Joe as "learning to move without tenseness." His focus was on using only the correct muscle to produce the movement.

Stamina: Joe indicated the need for endurance. He described muscular fatigue as one of the "poisons" to the body.

Review of Basic Pilates Mat Neutral Positions

Supine Neutral Alignment

The most important lesson that your clients will learn in Pilates is the ability to find and hold a neutral posture. This posture is easiest to achieve in the supine position and therefore should be one of the first positions in which you attempt to teach this concept. This position should be a precursor to all of the supine mat exercises, even though in many of the exercises, your clients will move in and out of supine neutral.

To position in neutral in the supine position, have your client begin by assuming a hook lying posture on the mat. The client should position his heels in line with his ischial tuberosities and his knees with his second toes. The anterior triangle of the pelvis should fall in the frontal plane in line with the ceiling and the floor. Another way to describe this position is to imagine the ischial tuberosities as headlights. The headlights should shine on the wall of the room and not on the ceiling.

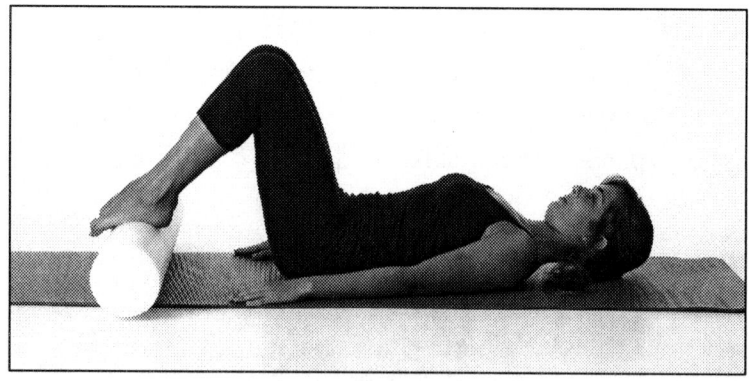

Supine Neutral Alignment

*Pilates, J., & Miller, W. (2000). In Gallagher, S., Kryzanowska, R. (Eds.), *The complete writings of Joseph H. Pilates.* Philadelphia, PA: BainBridgeBooks.

The 10th rib angle and ribcage should also lie in the frontal plane. In this position, the 11th and 12th ribs will lie on the mat. One way to visualize the proper position of the ribcage is to imagine the bottom opening of the ribs as a large light that will shine directly on the wall and not on the ceiling. When the ribs are drawn into the frontal plane, a participant with a short low back or lengthened abdomen may feel discomfort and challenge. If a client has difficulty maintaining the neutral pelvic position, try a proprioceptive pad under the coccyx (tailbone).

If a client has short lumbar extensor muscles, he may also experience cervical extension when achieving this position. If so, instruct the client to reach long out of the top back of his head, lengthening the back of the neck. If the client continues to demonstrate cervical extension, instruct him to place a small towel under his head for support. The towel can be gradually removed as the client gains length in the back extensors and flexibility in the front of the chest. Achieving this neutral position will be vital to the success of creating muscle balance through Pilates. Neutral postures should be reinforced with each and every lesson.

Prone Neutral Alignment

Finding neutral alignment in the prone position will be more challenging for most of the general population. People spend 90 percent of their days and nights in flexion, and the prone position requires extension of many of the joints. It will be even more difficult for older adults, due to changes in posture. Even though this position will be challenging, it is very important and should be continually encouraged.

To find neutral position in prone, instruct your client to lie face down on the mat with his hands under his forehead. Palms should be facing downward, and heels should be in line with the ischial tuberosities. Have the client position his pelvis so that the posterior triangle (PSIS and coccyx) is in line with the ceiling and the pubic bone is on the mat. Once these bony prominences are in place, the client should attempt

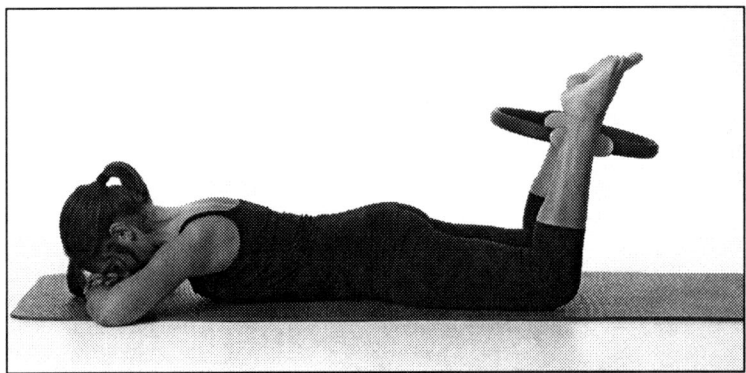

Prone Neutral Alignment

to draw the abdomen up and away from the floor, positioning the ribcage in the frontal plane. In the prone position, many will rest on the anterior 10th rib angles as if they were elbows. These boney prominences should only lightly touch the floor.

At times, many clients will raise the shoulder blades and shorten the neck in this position, so remind them to reach the top back of their head to the wall in front of them and to lengthen the back of their neck. If a client has shoulder problems, the prone position can be achieved with arms at the sides and a small towel roll under the forehead instead of the hands.

Seated Neutral Alignment

The long sit position used for seated exercise in Pilates builds a critical relationship in the muscles of the lumbopelvic area. These muscles frequently become imbalanced in the general population and often lead to back and hip problems. Two common populations affected are seniors and children. Seniors tend to sit on the floor less as they age, and children are affected in this area by rapid growth spurts. Learning and practicing the long sit position will maintain vital relationships between the muscles of the lumbopelvic complex.

For these reasons, teaching your clients how to find seated neutral alignment might be one of two of the most beneficial lessons. Pilates is most effective when practiced frequently, and both seated and standing alignment can be practiced continuously by anyone. Good posture does not simply come from exercise sessions; it comes from understanding where you should be and making a conscious effort to be there.

To find neutral position in sitting, have the client begin with the long sit position. Instruct the client to place the boney landmarks of the bike seat in the same plane as the floor. A good way to describe this position is to sit up on the ischial tuberosities or sitting bones and align the pubic bone (pubic ramus) with the floor. The legs should be as wide as the ischial tuberosities, and the knees should be straight with no rotation

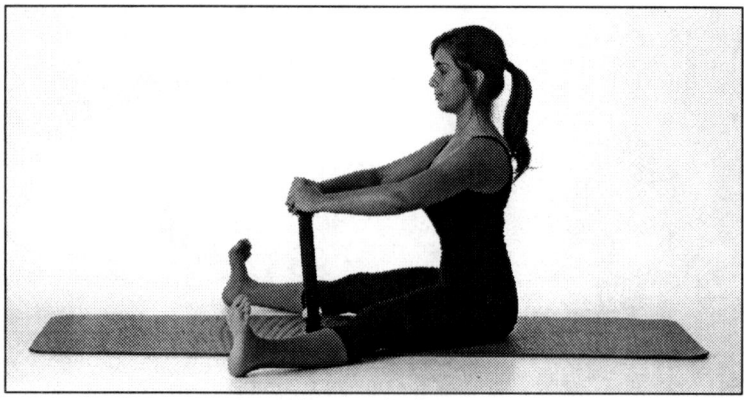

Seated Neutral Alignment

at the hip. The anterior part of the 10th rib should be in line with the anterior superior iliac spine (ASIS), and the shoulders should be lined up over the hips. The client should lengthen the neck and reach the top back of his head to the ceiling. He should open the chest, and keep the shoulders down.

If your client is unable to sit up on the bike seat with the legs fully extended, instruct him to position himself on a small box. This modification is preferable as it will encourage lengthening of the hamstrings which is needed to achieve supine neutral. If the knees are allowed to bend, the goal of balance between the hamstrings and hip flexors may never be achieved.

Side-Lying Neutral Alignment

For side-lying exercises, it is important to align the body in neutral to imitate the standing position. This alignment will create a stimulus for balanced muscle length from one side of the body to the other. It is important to work a muscle at the length in which it will perform its functional movement.

To find neutral in side lying, have the client align the torso with the mat and bring the legs slightly in front of him to take the pressure off the bursa of the hip. He should stack the hips as if lying in a hallway and reach the top leg longer than the bottom leg. Doing so will create a small unweighted area at the waist. Women with smaller waists may have an area of the waist that will not touch the floor. In men, this area will be less noticeable because of the size of their pelvis. Check to make sure that the anterior part of the 10th rib is in line with the ASIS. The shoulders should be open and relaxed, and the neck should be long.

Pilates offers many exercise options for side lying—including up/down, front/back, passé, bicycle, circles, hip adduction, and heal beats. The benefit of most of these versions of exercise is a balance of strength about the hip and core with an emphasis on the power and ability to engage the hip abductors.

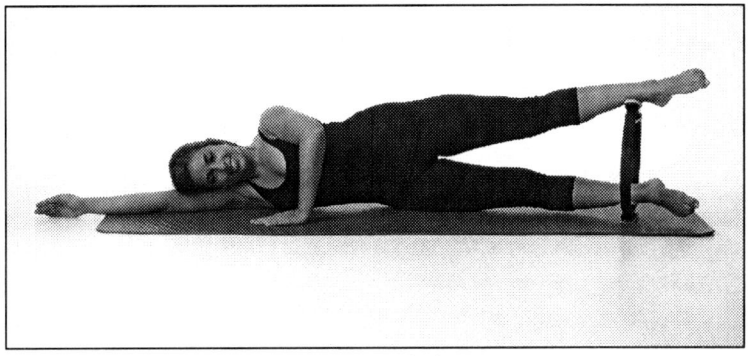

Side-Lying Neutral Alignment

For most instructors, the most common question from participants is: "How high should I lift my leg?" Instructors can confidently answer: "Lift the leg as high as you can without losing the neutral position of your torso." If the torso rolls backward, the emphasis of the work is placed on the hip flexor muscles. If the torso rolls forward, the emphasis is placed on the buttock muscles. If the space at the waist is diminished, the hip abductors, abdominals, and back extensors are worked at an inappropriate length. The height and repetitions of side-lying exercises should be directly controlled by the ability of the participant to maintain the neutral side-lying position.

By being attentive to alignment, you will know how much to encourage the height or swing of the leg, how many repetitions to perform, or when to progress to a more challenging version of the exercise. Watching alignment can become the answer to many of the questions that arise when performing Pilates mat work.

The Use of Props for Pilates Mat Work

Joseph Pilates invented several apparatuses to teach his method of Contrology. Today, practitioners use the reformer, Cadillac, wunda chair, pedi-pole, foot corrector, ladder barrel, low barrel, the circle (ring), and the tower. These apparatuses were used by Joseph Pilates to teach and perfect the movement in combination with the mat program. Today, many instructors do not have these apparatuses available, or they work in large groups where the use of the apparatus is not possible. In response to this need, many teachers continue to use the small props that Joseph Pilates created, including the circle or ring, the spine corrector, and the baby arc, or they attempt to simulate the effect of the other apparatuses with the foam roller.

This book will explore the use of the ring, the spine corrector, the baby arc, and the foam roller as teaching tools in the study of movement. These tools will be used in the following three ways:

- *To motivate and challenge the client.* When participants master a movement, they may become complacent and bored. Props such as the foam roller and the ring can make exercises more challenging and change their effect to hold the interest of the client.

- *To reinforce and support the client.* When participants are just beginning the mat work, they often need support to prevent injury to their spine or added reinforcement to maintain the proper alignment for safety.

- *To inform the client.* Participants often need direction or an impetus for proper movement. A prop such as the ring or the foam roller can assist with movement when a cue to move or compress the prop is provided by the instructor. This effect works much like a visual cue, but also provides a proprioceptive effect.

Choosing the Props

Rings

When choosing a Pilates ring, look for one that has handles on both the inside and the outside of the ring. Look for one with padded handles as it helps to keep the ring in place and is more comfortable on the skin. The resistance of the ring should be light, as the goal is never to squeeze the ring with all of your might. Basically, the participant needs to be able to hold the ring with his deep muscles without engaging the large muscles. Some rings are weighted, which can be useful as a client progresses.

Rollers

Many types of foam rollers are available, from the basic white foam to more advanced foams. The basic white foam roller is inexpensive and light, but not as durable. It will last only two to three months under heavy use. The more expensive foams are more durable, lasting years, and are often softer and more comfortable to lie on. Air rollers are also available. They are a lot like a Swiss ball in the shape of a roll. Air rollers are useful for clients with osteoporosis as they are soft and will not cause stress to their spines. The air rollers are also softer for clients who are tender when they lie on the roller.

Spine Corrector

The spine corrector is sometimes called the low barrel or the half barrel. When choosing a spine corrector, look for a steep barrel with a sharp angled seat. This shape is necessary to support the pelvis for many of the exercises. Be sure that the handles on the sides are comfortable and that they have a way to adjust the location of the handle for different size clients.

Baby Arc

The baby arc is a smaller version of the spine corrector without the seat. It is useful for smaller people, including women and children.

2

The Foam Roller

Articulating Bridge With One Roller

Category: Lower-body and core strengthening; spinal flexibility

Benefits: This exercise will increase spinal flexibility, and strengthen the abdominal, gluteal, and lower-back muscles.

Set-Up: Lie supine and position the roller horizontally at your feet. Place your feet on the roller aligning your heels with your ischial tuberosities and your knee caps with your second toes. Position your pelvis in neutral. Place your arms at your sides, and reach your fingers toward the roller. This positioning will assist in drawing your shoulders down.

Movement: While keeping the roller still, posteriorly tilt your pelvis, and begin to peel your spine from the mat one vertebra at a time. Continue to lift until your anterior superior iliac spine (ASIS) is aligned with your 10th rib angle. Then begin to descend one vertebra at a time back to the supine position. Think of returning with the highest thoracic vertebra to the mat first.

Cues:

- Keep the roller still as you articulate up and down.
- Do not bridge onto your neck.
- Keep your shoulders down, and lengthen your neck.
- Do not allow your knees to move in or out during the movement.
- Keep the weight to the inside of your feet.

Modification: Limit the motion, and perform just a posterior pelvic tilt.

Progression: While in the lifted position, lift one leg off the roller, keeping the roller still and maintaining neutral alignment.

Breathing: Inhale to prepare, and exhale as you lift. Inhale at the top, and exhale as you return to the starting position.

Repetitions: 5 to 8

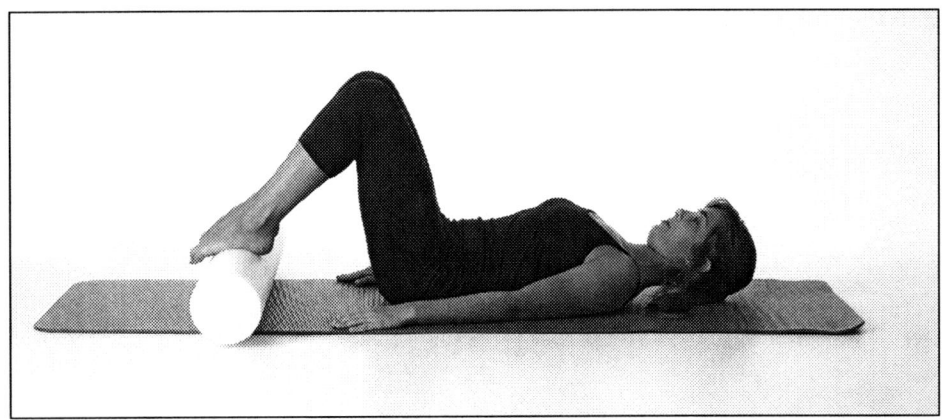

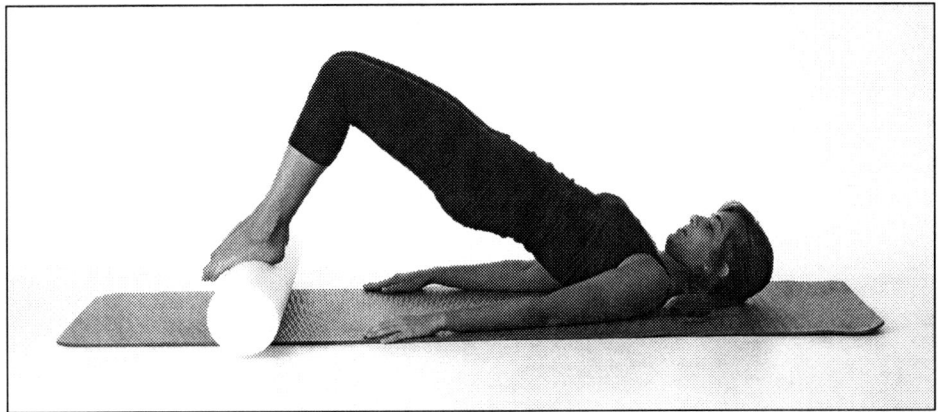

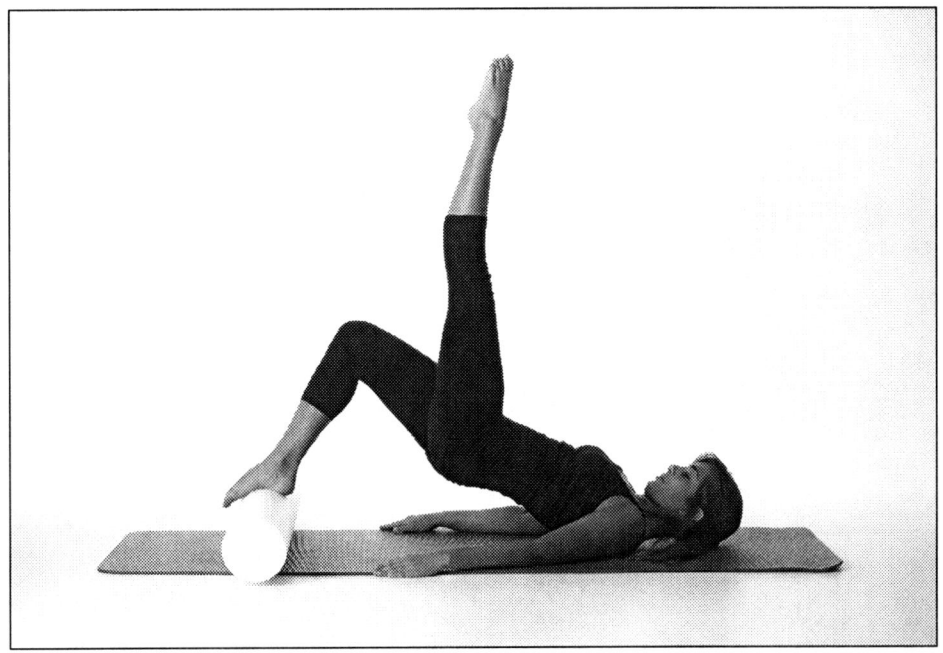

21

Articulating Bridge With Two Rollers

Category: Lower-body and core strengthening; spinal flexibility

Benefits: This exercise will increase spinal flexibility and strengthen the abdominal, gluteal, and lower-back muscles.

Set-Up: Lie supine with your head and spine on one foam roller. Place your feet on the second roller, aligning your heels with your ischial tuberosities. Position your pelvis and ribcage in neutral, and reach long out of the top back of your head.

Movement: While keeping the roller at your feet still, posteriorly tilt your pelvis, and begin to peel your spine from the roller one vertebra at a time. Continue to lift until your ASIS is aligned with your 10th rib angle. Then begin to descend one vertebra at a time back to the supine position on the roller.

Cues:

- Keep the rollers still as you articulate up and down.
- Do not bridge onto your neck.
- Keep your shoulders down, and lengthen your neck.
- Do not allow your knees to move out or in during the movement.
- Keep the weight to the inside of your feet.

Modification: Perform the exercise with only one roller under your spine and head. Keep your knees bent with your feet on the floor.

Progression: While in the bridge position, lift one leg off the roller, keeping the roller still and maintaining alignment.

Breathing: Inhale to prepare, and exhale as you lift. Inhale at the top, and exhale as you return to the starting position.

Repetitions: 5 to 8

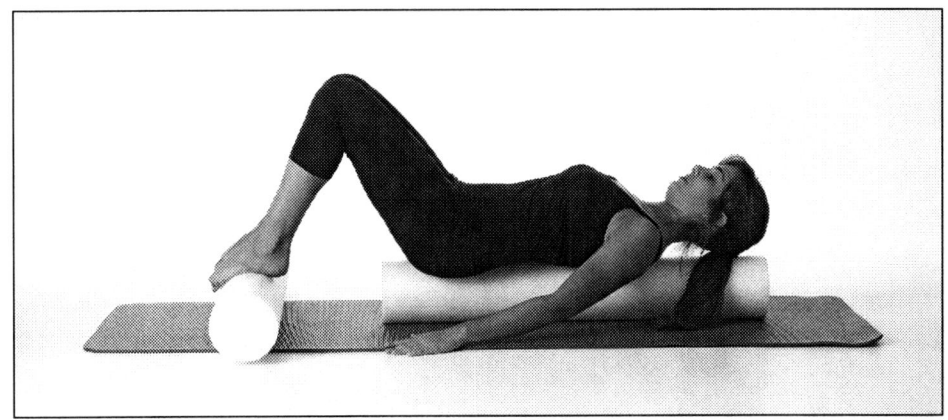

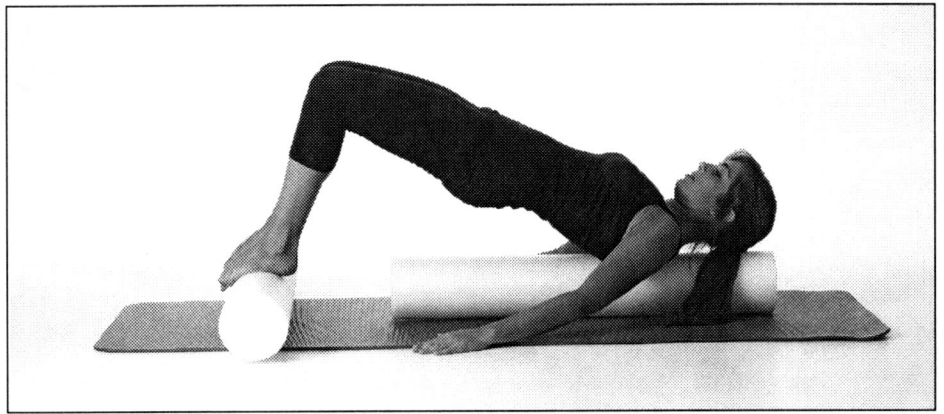

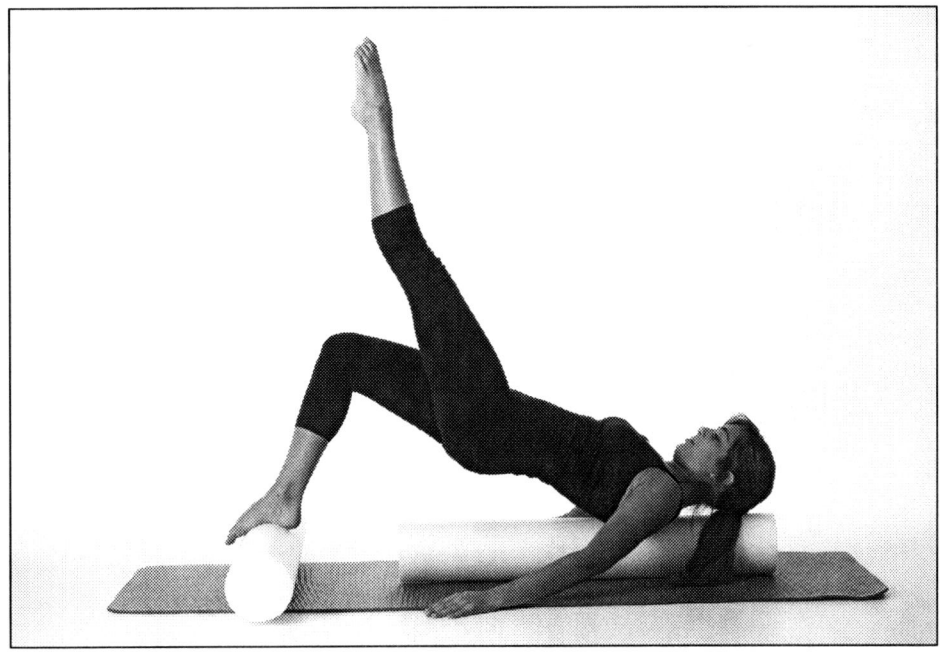

Leg Circles

Category: Lower-body and core strengthening

Benefits: This exercise will strengthen the hip flexors and lengthen the iliotibial band and hamstrings.

Set-Up: Lie with your spine and head on the roller and feet on the floor with your knees bent. Extend your arms along your sides, and touch the floor to assist with balance. Position your pelvis and ribcage in neutral, and lengthen the back of your neck. Extend one leg toward the ceiling, and slightly rotate your hip outward.

Movement: While keeping the roller still, circle your leg down toward the mat, crossing the midline of your body, and then bring it around to the starting position. The emphasis should be on the upswing of the movement. Try to keep a neutral pelvis during the movement, and increase the size of the circle only when you gain the ability to maintain pelvic neutral. After three to five circles in one direction, reverse the direction of the circles. Flex the leg into your chest to stretch before repeating the exercise with the opposite leg.

Cues:

- Keep your roller stable and your spine and pelvis neutral as your leg circles.
- Maintain the position of the hip in outward rotation or in neutral as you circle.

Progression: Extend the bottom leg along the floor or place the bottom leg on the ring or a small ball.

Breathing: Inhale as you begin to circle your leg, and exhale as you bring it back to the starting position.

Repetitions: 3 to 5 circles in each direction

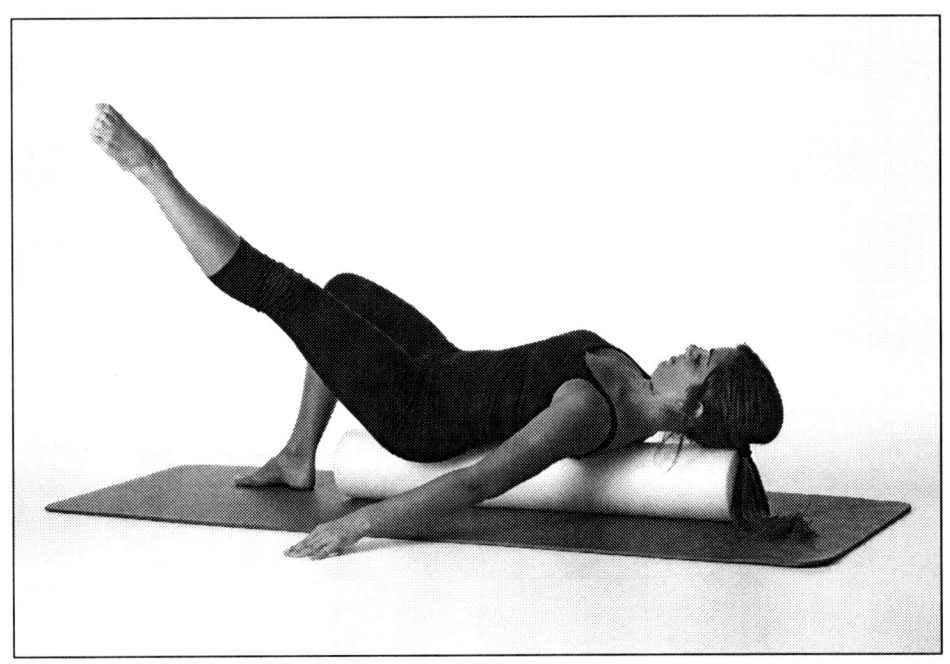

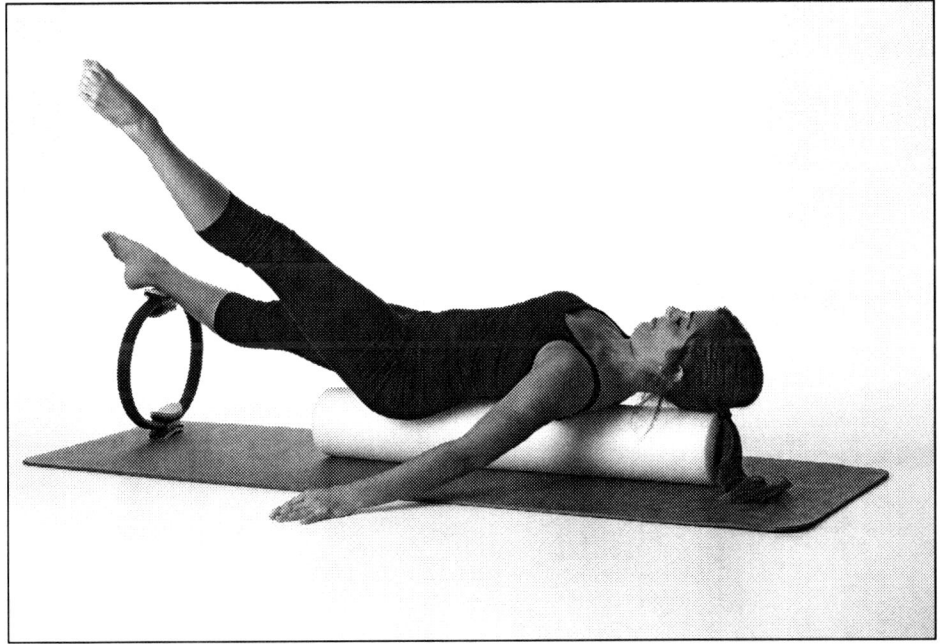

Roll-Up on Two Rollers

Category: Core strengthening; hip and spine flexibility

Benefits: This exercise will strengthen the abdominal muscles and increase the length of the spine extensors and hip extensors.

Set-Up: Lie with your spine and back on one roller and your legs extended on the second roller. Position the pelvis and spine in neutral. Extend your arms over your head while keeping your ribs in line with your pelvis. Point your toes softly, and outwardly rotate your legs into a Pilates "V."

Movement: Slowly curl your head and shoulders off the roller, keeping both rollers still. Flex your spine forward into a "C" curve as you reach toward your feet. Flex your feet, and maintain the "C" curve as you return your spine to the roller one vertebra at a time.

Cues:

- On the way down, look through your hands like a camera.
- Keep your shoulders down and back throughout the exercise.
- Reach through the crown of your head as you flex the spine.
- Reach your ischial tuberosities toward your heels throughout the movement.

Breathing: Inhale deeply before beginning the movement, and then exhale as you roll up. Pause in the seated position to inhale, and exhale as you roll back down to the roller.

Modification: Do the roll-down movement only. Roll on your side to come up, and then reposition for the next repetition.

Repetitions: 5 to 8

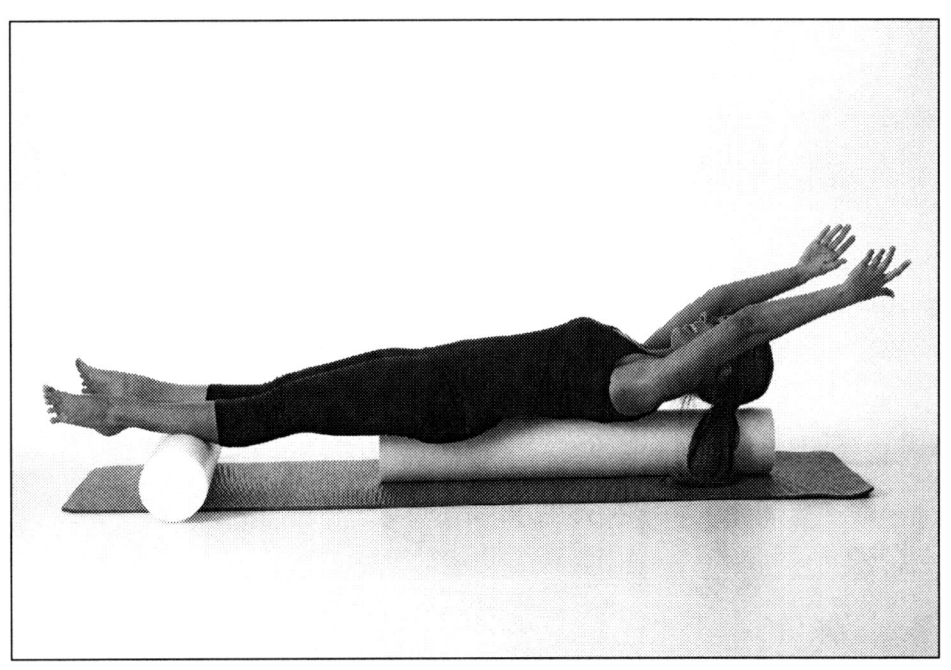

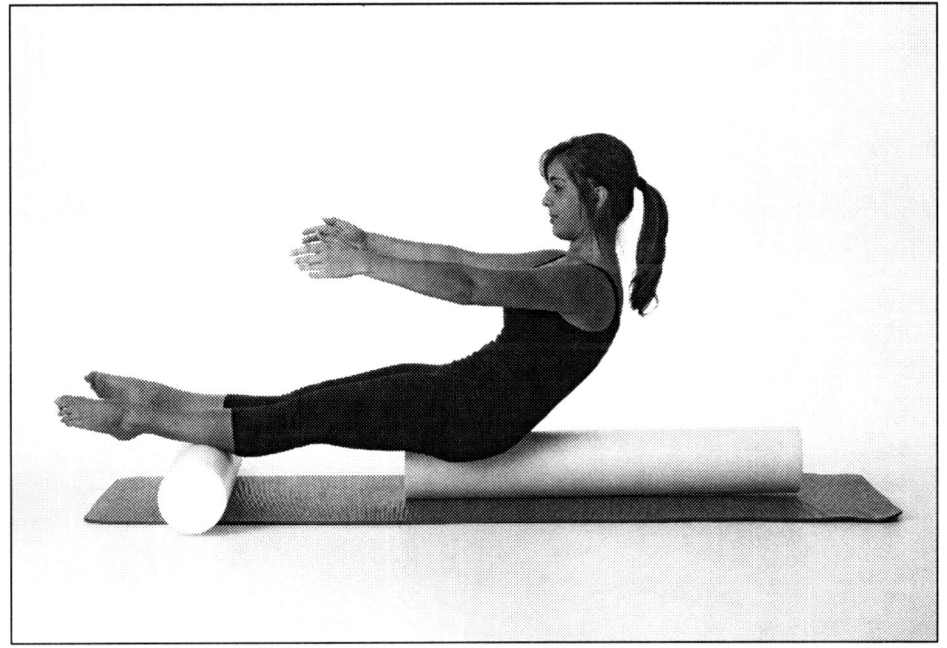

Hundred With Two Rollers

Category: Core strengthening and lumbar flexibility

Benefits: This exercise will strengthen the abdominal muscles and lengthen the spine extensors.

Set-Up: Place two rollers in a "T." Lie with your head and spine on one roller, and place your feet on the second roller. Position your spine and pelvis in neutral, and line up your heels with your ischial tuberosities. Place your arms at your side with your palms down.

Movement: Slowly curl up to a position where you can hold neutral pelvis. Reach your fingers toward your feet, drawing your shoulders down your back. While maintaining a stable torso, move your arms up and down as if you were slapping water.

Cues:

- Keep both rollers still during the arm movement.
- Keep your shoulders down and back throughout the exercise.
- Reach through the crown of your head as you flex the spine.

Modification: Remove one of the rollers, and place either your back or your feet on the floor.

Breathing: Inhale as your prepare, and exhale as you roll up. Then, continue breathing in sets of five inhalations and five exhalations.

Repetitions: 30 to 100 (3 sets of 10; 10 sets of 10)

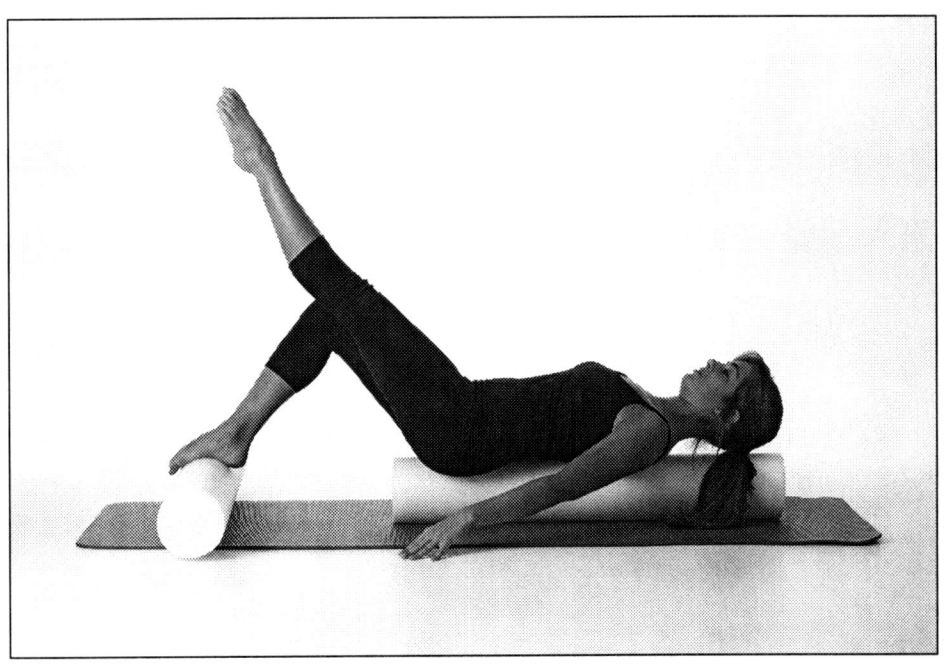
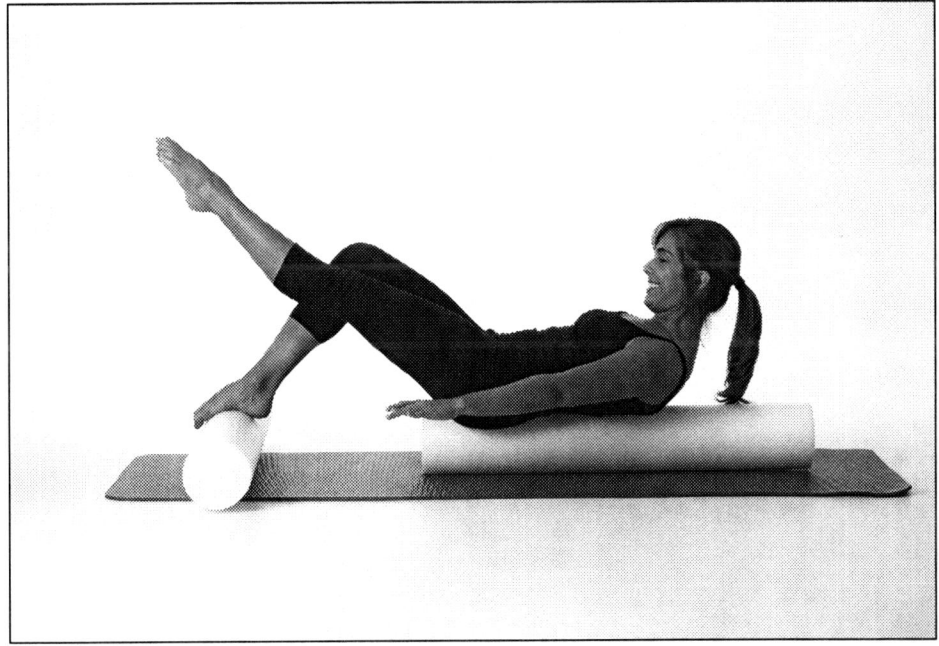

Ribcage Arms on Two Rollers

Category: Core strengthening and stability

Benefits: This exercise will strengthen the core and improves balance.

Set-Up: Lie with your head and spine on one roller and your feet on another roller. Your spine and pelvis should be in neutral position, and your feet should be in line with your ischial tuberosities. Extend your arms toward the ceiling.

Movement: While maintaining neutral pelvis and spine, raise both of your arms over your head, and lift one leg to the tabletop position. Maintain your knee-to-second-toe alignment. Return to the starting position, and repeat with your other leg. Continue to alternate your legs for the desired repetitions. Avoid crossing the midline of your body as you lift your leg.

Cues:

- Reach long through the crown of your head as you extend your arms.
- Keep your ribs aligned with your pelvis as the arms move.
- Keep the roller still and stable as you perform the movement.
- Keep your pelvis neutral as your leg lifts.

Modification: Remove the roller under your feet, and place them on the floor.

Progression: Raise the opposite arm and leg in opposition to one another, or try these movements with your eyes closed.

Breathing: Inhale as you prepare to move, and exhale as you perform the movement.

Repetitions: 5 to 8

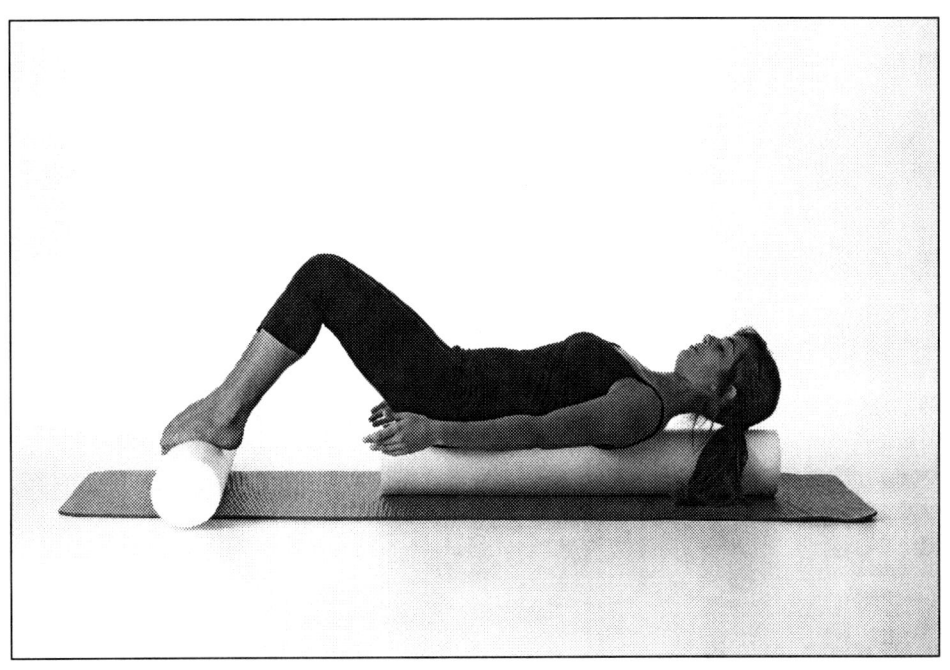

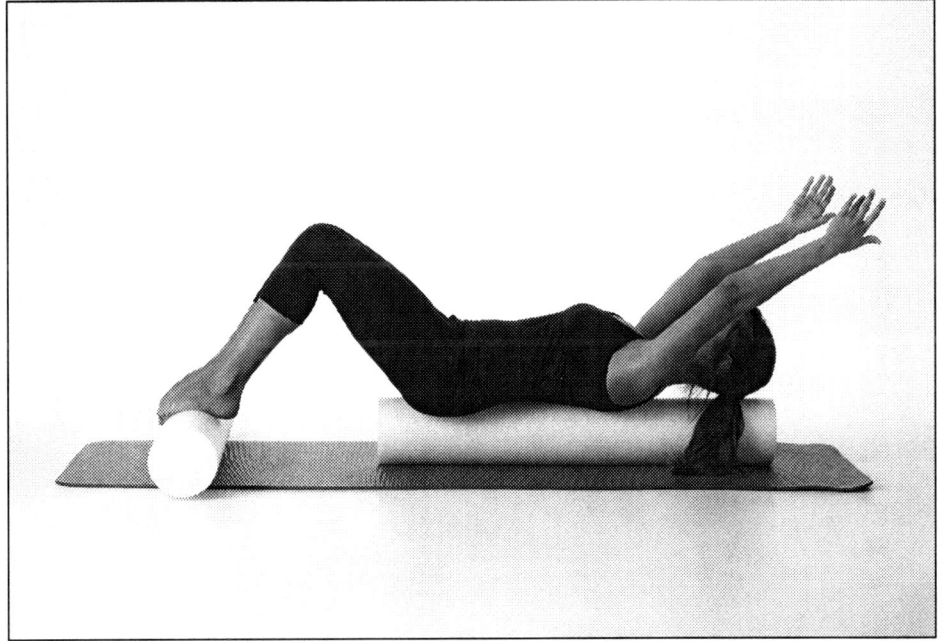

Scissors

Category: Lower-body and core strengthening; lower-body flexibility

Benefits: This exercise will strengthen the pelvic floor while lengthening the hamstrings, hip flexors, and spine extensors.

Set-Up: Lie with your back on the mat and your pelvis posteriorly tilted on the foam roller. Your lumbar spine should be in flexion, and your ischial tuberosities should point upward. Hold the roller in place with your hands.

Movement: Extend both legs up at an angle in which you can still maintain flexion of the lumbar spine. Extend one leg over head and one leg toward the floor. Be sure to keep the knees straight and the ASIS in line. Do not let the pelvis rock from side to side as you alternate slowly for the desired repetitions.

Cues:

- Keep your knees and second toes aligned.
- Reach your ischial tuberosity to the opposite inner thigh to maintain pelvic alignment.

Progression: Bend the knee of the leg toward the floor for a deeper stretch of the hip flexor.

Breathing: Inhale to begin, and exhale as you extend your legs. Inhale and exhale as you switch leg position.

Repetitions: 5 to 8

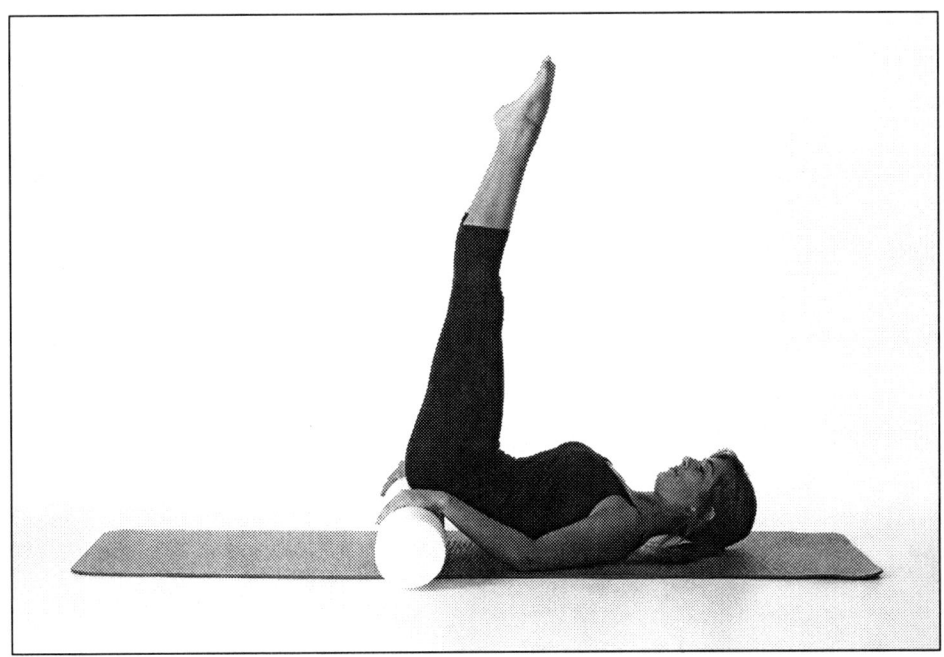
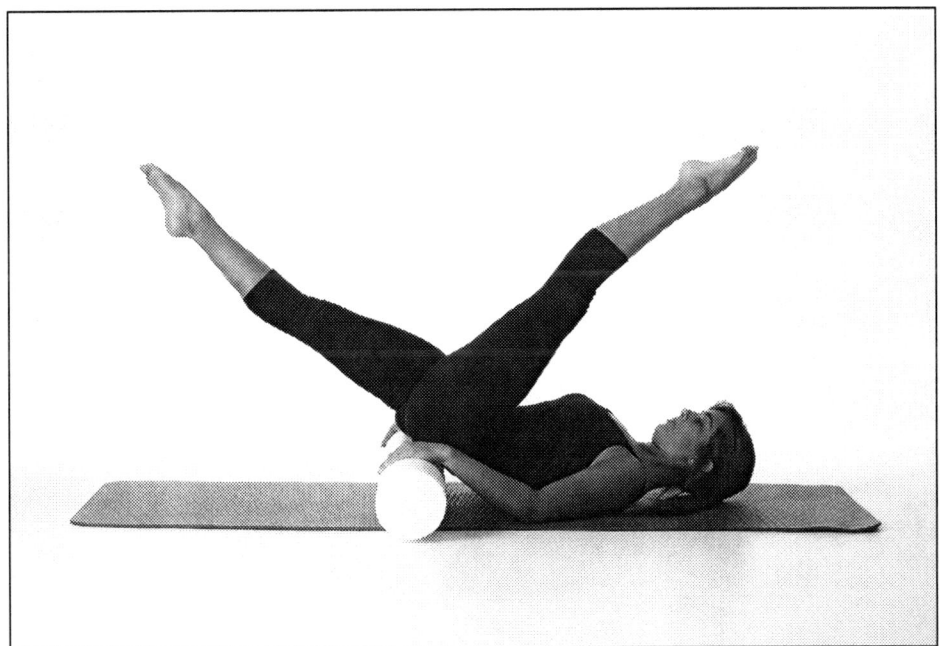

Helicopter

Category: Lower-body and core strengthening; lower-body flexibility

Benefits: This exercise will strengthen the pelvic floor while lengthening the hamstrings, hip flexors, hip adductors, and spine extensors.

Set-Up: Lie with your back on the mat and your pelvis posteriorly tilted on the foam roller. Your lumbar spine should be in flexion, and your ischial tuberosities should point upward. Hold the roller in place with your hands.

Movement: Extend both legs up at an angle in which you can still maintain flexion of the lumbar spine. Extend one leg over your head and one leg toward the floor. Be sure to keep the knees straight and the ASIS in line. Do not let the pelvis rock from side to side as you rotate your hips to move into a straddle position. Circle your legs around to the opposite split position, and then return to the straddle. Continue this movement for the desired repetitions.

Cues:

- Keep your knees and second toes aligned.
- Reach your ischial tuberosity to the opposite inner thigh to maintain pelvic alignment.
- Move slowly, and hold the stretch.

Breathing: Inhale to begin, and exhale as you extend your legs. Inhale and exhale as you switch leg position.

Repetitions: 5 to 8

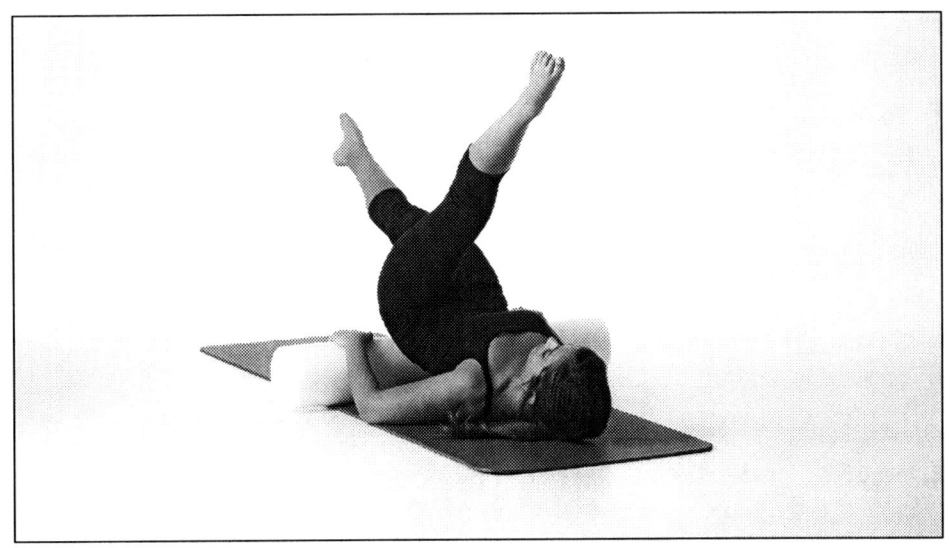

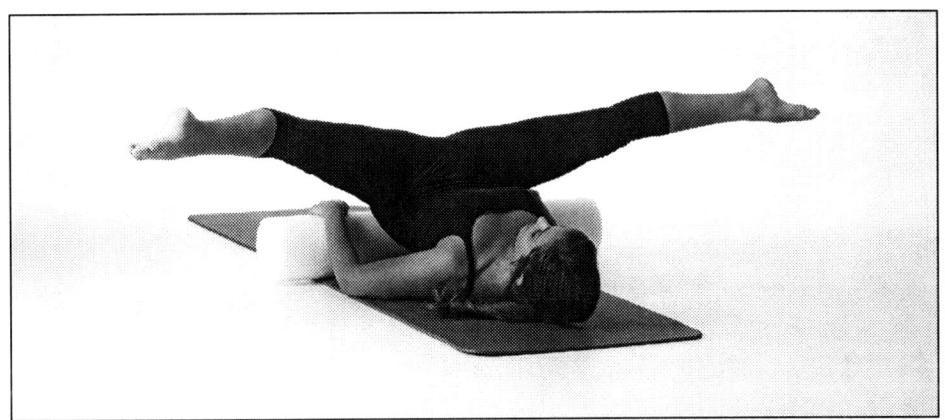

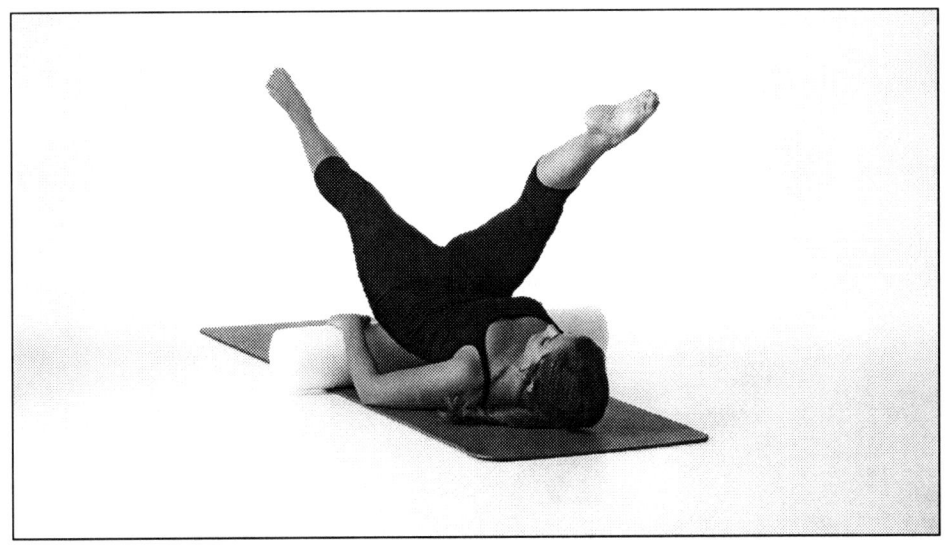

Mermaid

Category: Spine and hip flexibility

Benefits: This exercise will lengthen the quadratus lumborum and hip muscles. It also will strengthen the quadratus lumborum and the abdominal obliques.

Set-Up: Sit mermaid-style with one hip internally rotated and the other hip externally rotated. Reach your ischial tuberosities to the floor, and align your pelvis and ribcage with the wall in front of you. Place the roller slightly in front of you on the side of the front leg with your hand on the top.

Movement: Round your spine in a "C" curve to the side as you roll the roller away from you. Keep your shoulder stable, and control the roller. Once you have reached your limit, draw the roller back to the set-up position.

Cues:

- Keep your torso square with the wall in front of you as you move.
- Lift your spine up and away from the floor without lifting your pelvis.
- Keep your shoulders down as your roll the roller.

Modifications: If you are unable to sit in mermaid position, sit on a small box.

Variation: While rounded to the side toward the roller, rotate the spine and place the other hand on the roller. Stay rotated, and extend into a flat back position. The roller will roll toward you as you extend your spine.

Breathing: Inhale to prepare, and exhale as you round your spine toward the roller. For the swan variation, you can inhale as the spine extends to help lengthen the spine.

Repetitions: 5 to 8 on each side

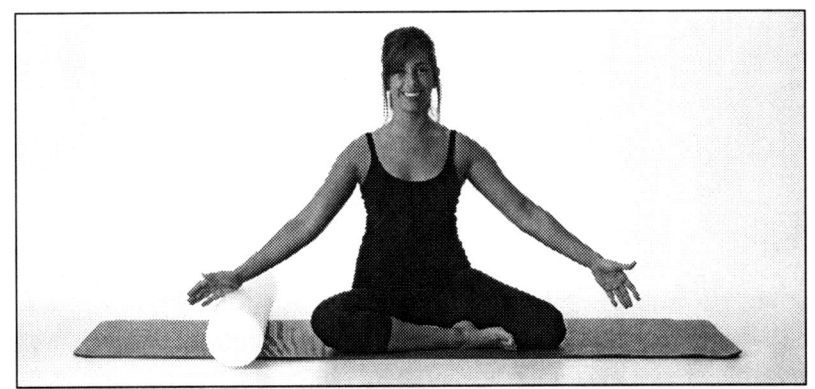
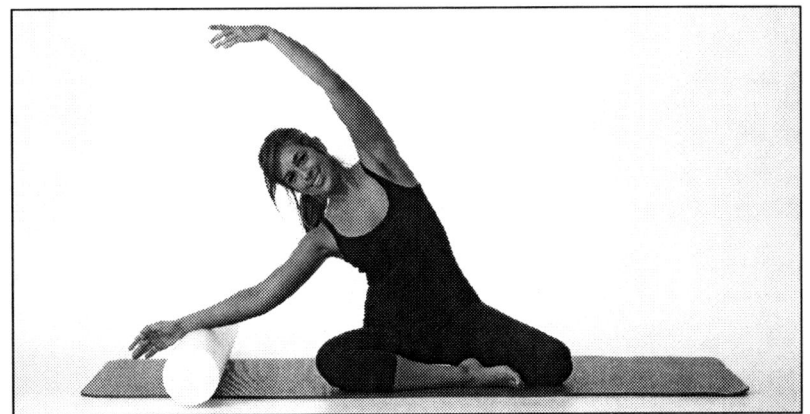
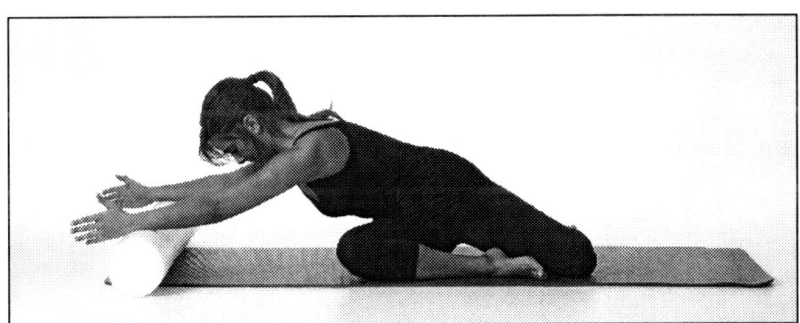
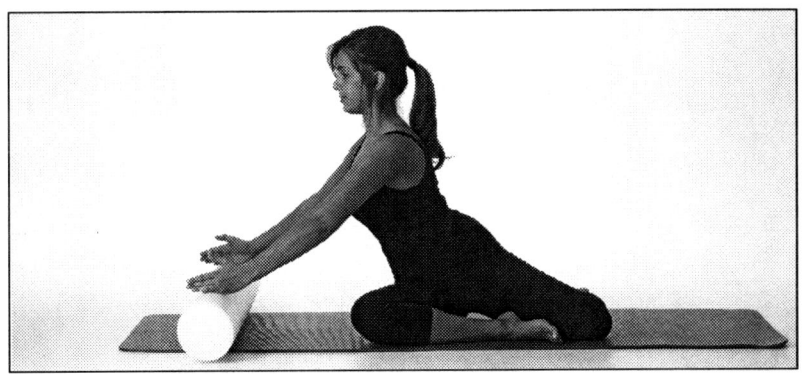

Hip Abductor

Category: Lower-body strengthening and flexibility; core strengthening and stability

Benefits: This exercise will strengthen the hip adductor and abductor muscles while lengthening the iliotibial band. Maintaining the neutral alignment will also challenge core stability.

Set-Up: Lie in side-lying neutral alignment with your bottom leg bent at the knee and your top leg resting on the foam roller. For side-lying neutral alignment, line your back up with the mat and place your legs slightly in front of you. Stack your hips and shoulders, and reach your top leg long to line up your pelvis in the transverse plane. The roller will roll slightly away from you as you reach your top leg long. Rest your head on your lower arm, and use the top arm for balance.

Movement: While in neutral alignment, roll the roller away with your top leg. Lift the leg off the roller in outward rotation, and then return to the roller. Finish by rolling the roller back toward you. Repeat for the desired repetitions.

Cues:

- Keep your hips stacked.
- Keep your shoulders down, stacked, and open.
- Reach long out of your legs.

Progression: Lift your upper body off the floor to rest onto your forearm.

Variation: Roll the roller away with the top leg, and maintain this position as you perform adduction of the bottom leg.

Breathing: Inhale to begin, and exhale on the movement.

Repetitions: 5 to 8 on each side

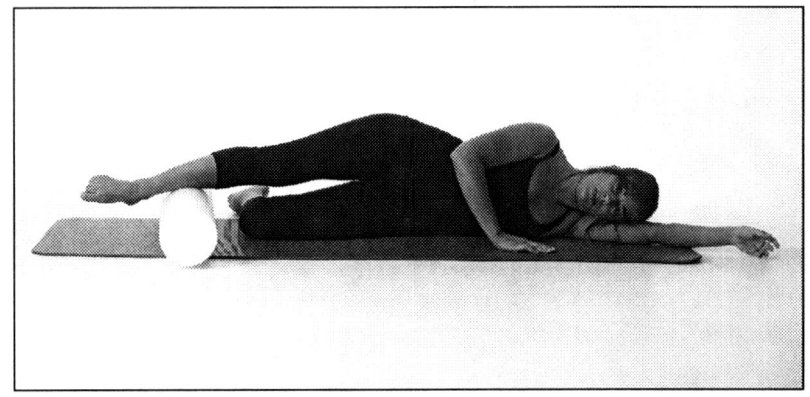
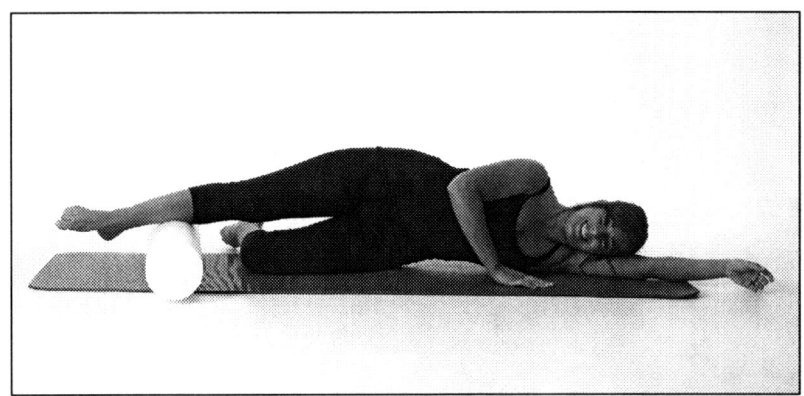
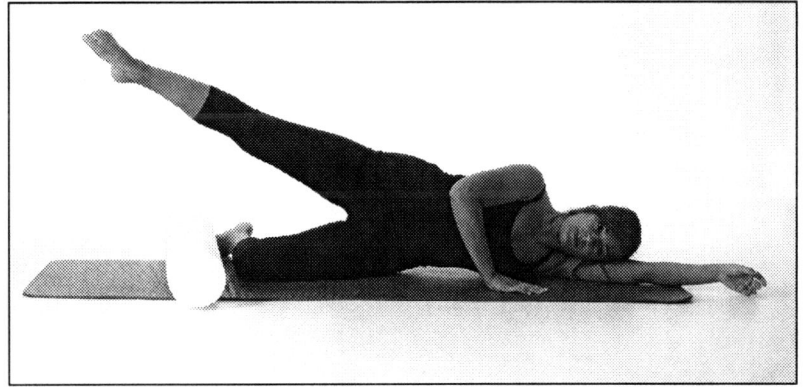
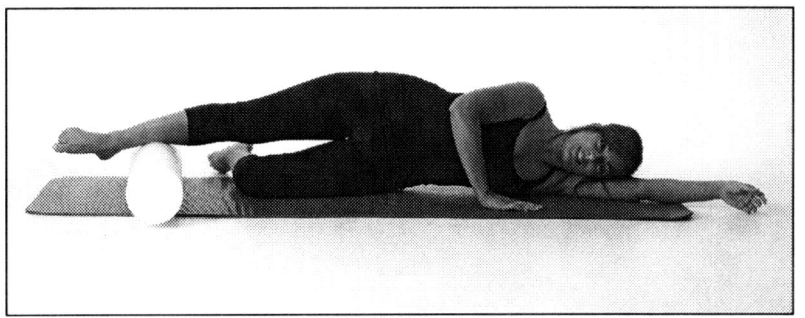

39

Eve's Lunge

Category: Lower-body flexibility; balance; core stability

Benefits: This exercise will lengthen the hip flexors and improve balance and coordination. It will also strengthen the core and lower extremities.

Set-Up: Stand with your feet hip-width apart and the roller lying horizontally behind you. Place the top of one foot on the roller, and bend the knee of your supporting leg. Position your pelvis in neutral and your knee over your second toe.

Movement: Reach the leg that is on the roller back, and roll the roller away from you. Keep the knee of the supporting leg aligned with your second toe. Use the leg on the roller to draw the roller beneath you while maintaining neutral alignment in your pelvis and upper body. Repeat for the desired repetitions.

Cues:

- Reach through the crown of your head to lengthen your neck.
- Keep the foot of the supporting leg from rolling in or out.
- Keep your ribs aligned with your ASIS.

Modification: Hold onto a chair or pole for support.

Breathing: Inhale to begin, and exhale as you press the roller back. Inhale when the leg is extended, and exhale as you draw the leg back to the beginning position.

Repetitions: 5 to 8 on each side

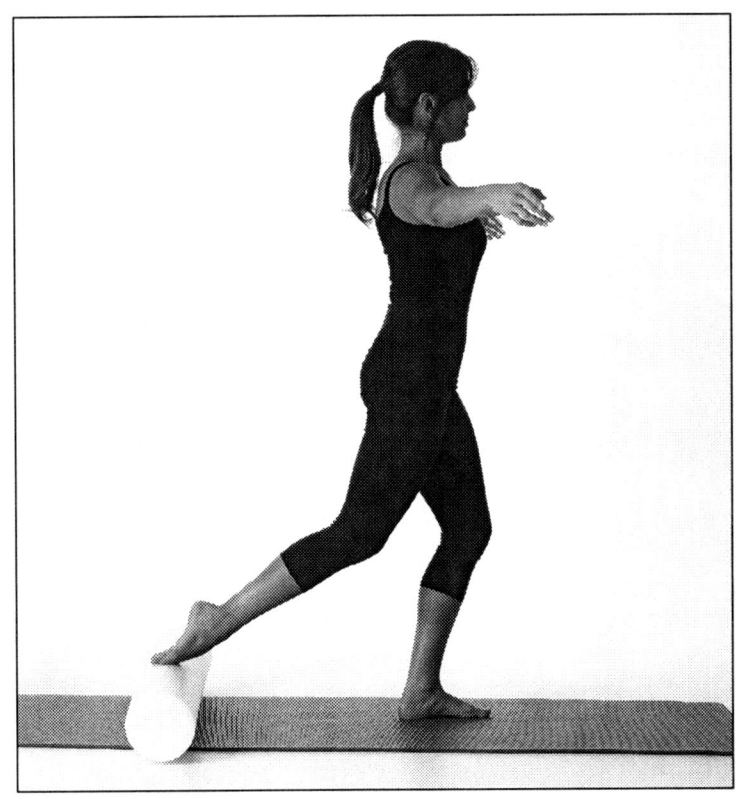
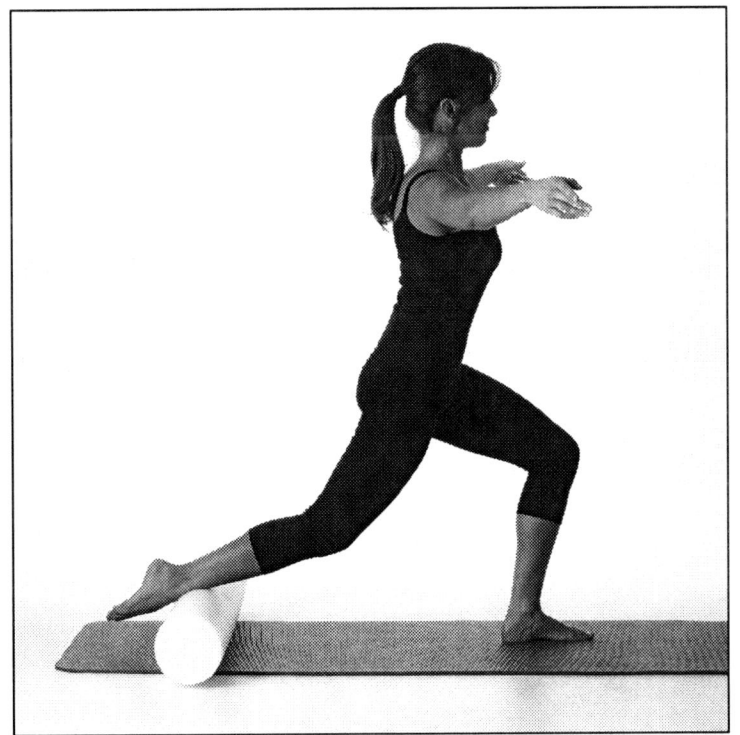

Knee Stretch (Abdominal Tuck) on Two Rollers

Category: Lower-body and spinal flexibility; core strengthening

Benefits: This exercise will lengthen the back extensors and strengthen the abdominal muscles.

Set-Up: Place two rollers side-by-side. Kneel on one roller, and place your forearms on the other. Posteriorly tilt your pelvis and round your spine into flexion.

Movement: Draw both rollers toward each other by drawing your knees toward your elbows. Imagine rounding your spine into a "C" curve from your head to tailbone. Hold and stretch the spine before moving back to the beginning position.

Cues:

- Reach long through the crown of your head to lengthen your spine.
- Keep your shoulders down your back.
- Avoid pulling the rollers with your arms and legs.

Modification: Remove the roller under your forearms, and place your hands on the floor.

Breathing: Inhale to begin, and exhale as the rollers draw together.

Repetitions: 3 to 5

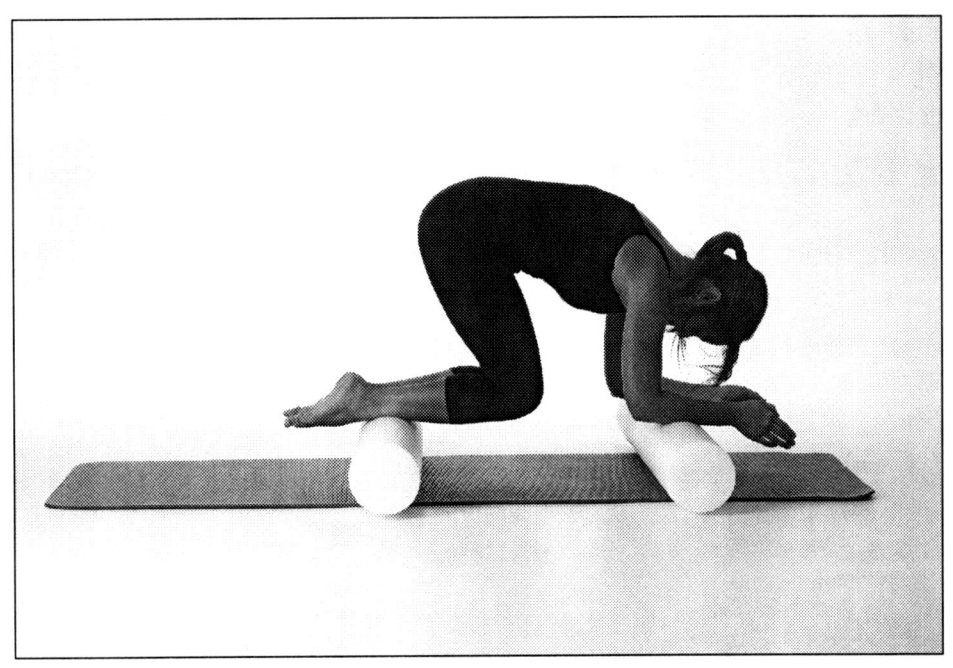

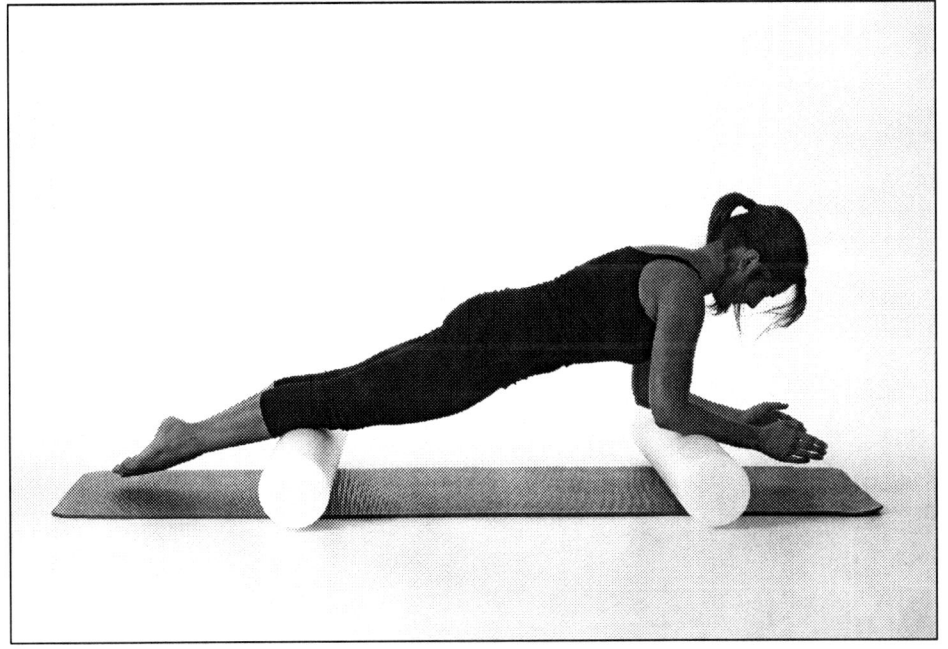

Knee Stretch (Abdominal Tuck) on One Roller

Category: Spinal flexibility; core and upper-body strengthening

Benefits: This exercise will lengthen the spine extensors and strengthen the abdominal muscles. It also has an effect on the upper core by increasing the stability of the shoulder girdle.

Set-Up: Place a roller behind you, and position your hands on the floor directly beneath your shoulders. Extend one leg behind you with the top of your foot resting on the roller. Add the second leg as you lift into a plank position. Your pelvis, spine, and shoulder girdle should be in neutral alignment.

Movement: Draw your knees toward your chest while keeping your arms directly beneath your shoulders. Your spine will round into a "C" curve. Return to the starting position, and repeat for the desired repetitions.

Cues:

- Keep a wide back, and watch for "winging" shoulder blades.
- Reach long through the crown of your head.
- Draw your navel to your spine as you round into the "C" curve.

Modifications:

- If you are unable to fully extend your legs, limit the range of motion by placing only your knees on the roller.
- If you have weak wrists, place either a rolled-up mat or towel beneath the heel of your hand to limit wrist extension.

Breathing: Inhale to prepare, and exhale as your draw the roller under you. Inhale in the round position, and then exhale to return to the plank position.

Repetitions: 3 to 5

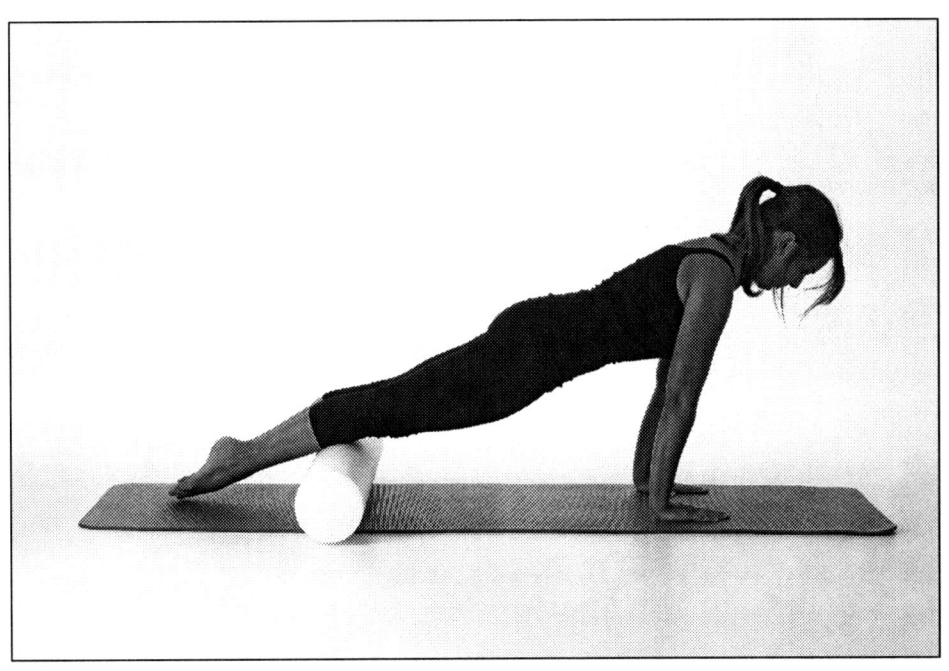

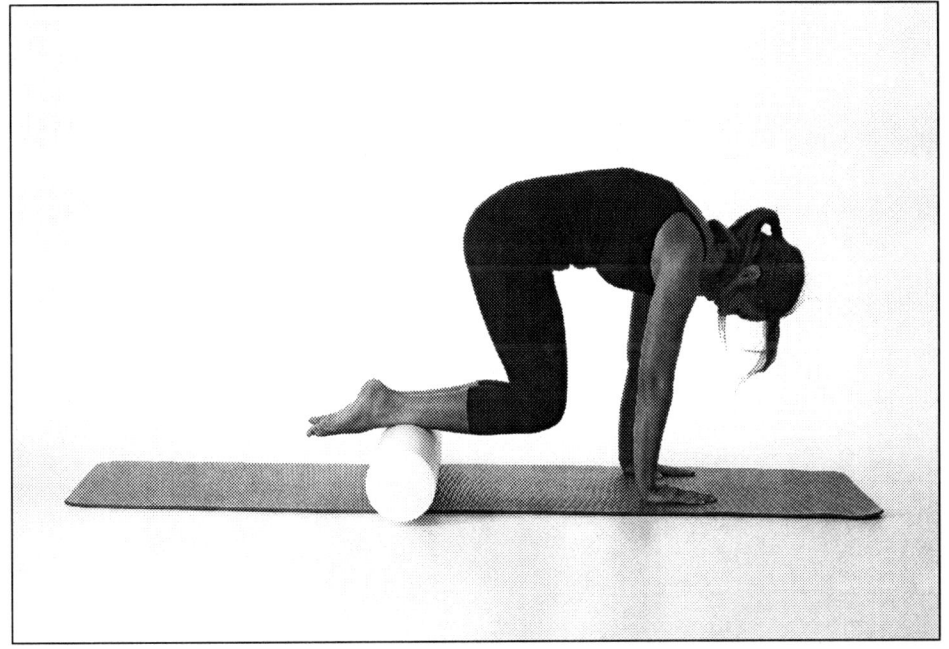

Modified Swimming on Two Rollers

Category: Core strengthening and stability

Benefits: This exercise will strengthen the back and core muscles and improve balance.

Set-Up: Kneel on one roller with your knees directly beneath your hips. Place your hands on the second roller with your hands directly beneath your shoulders. Position your spine and pelvis in neutral alignment.

Movement: While maintaining neutral spine, reach the opposite arm and leg. Repeat on the other side and continue for the desired repetitions.

Cues:

- Keep your back wide and shoulders down.
- Lift your arms and legs *only* as high as you can while keeping neutral alignment.
- Reach through the crown of your head to lengthen your neck.
- Avoid twisting your torso as you perform the movement.

Modification: Remove one of the rollers, and place either your hands or knees on the floor.

Breathing: Inhale to prepare, and exhale as you reach your arm and leg.

Repetitions: 5 to 8 on each side

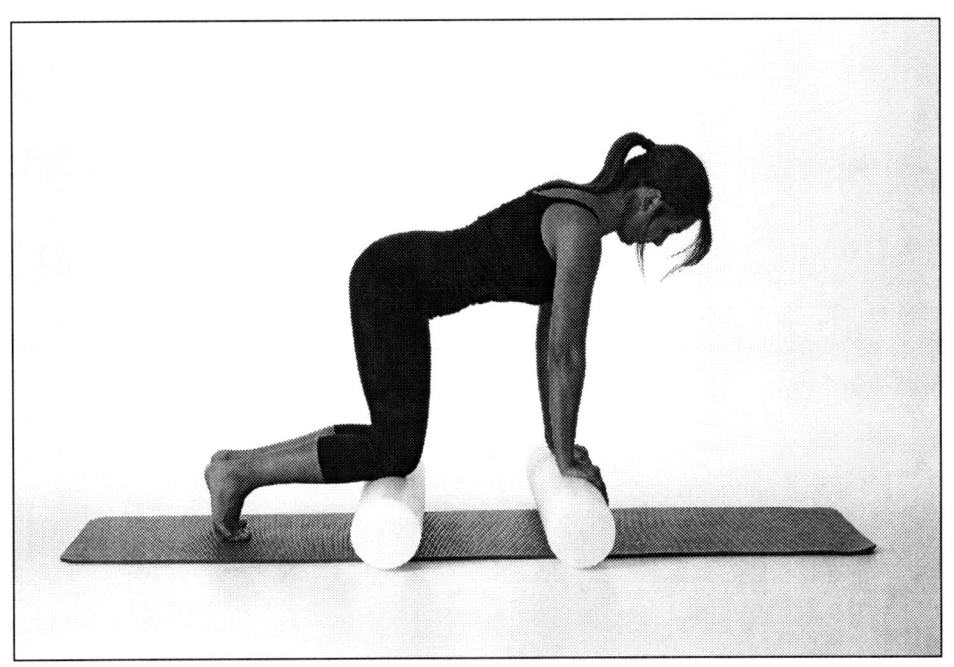

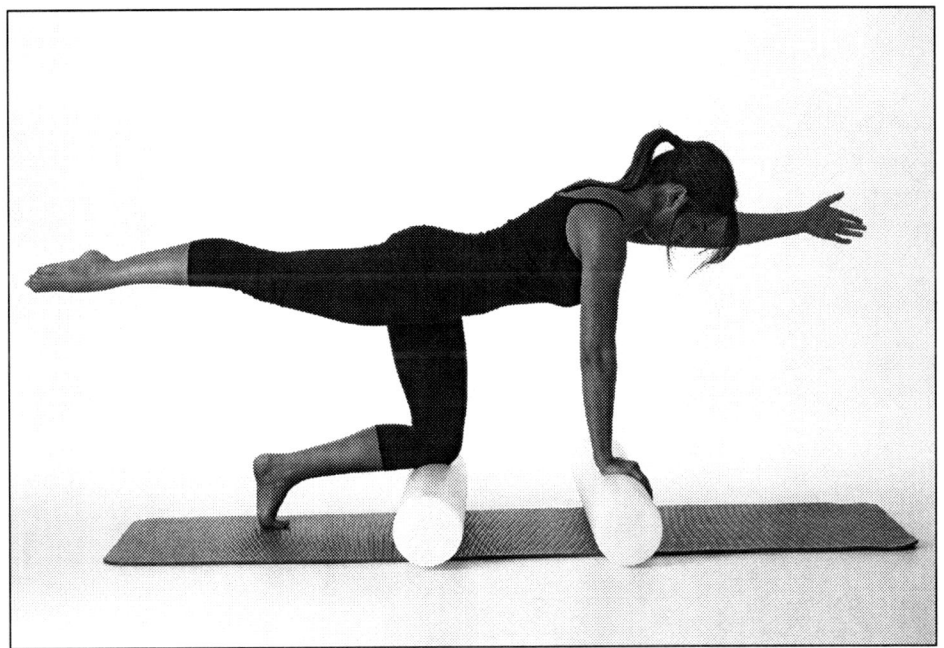

Push-Up With Hands on the Roller

Category: Core and upper-body strengthening

Benefits: This exercise will strengthen the muscles of the arms, chest, and back, and it will improve the stability of the core.

Set-Up: Place your hands on the roller with your thumbs and fingers pointing forward. Align your hands directly beneath your shoulders. Extend both legs behind you hip-width apart with the balls of your feet on the floor. Position your spine and pelvis in neutral alignment.

Movement: While maintaining neutral alignment, bring your upper body toward the roller by bending your elbows. Pause at the bottom of the movement, and then return to the beginning position. Continue for the desired repetitions.

Cues:

- Reach long through the crown of your head.
- Keep your back wide and chest open.
- Keep your spine in neutral alignment as you perform the movement.
- Avoid hyperextension of your elbows.

Modification: If you are a beginning participant, place your knees on the floor in a modified push-up position, or just limit the range of motion of the push-up.

Breathing: Inhale to prepare, and exhale as you lower toward the floor. Inhale as you pause at the bottom of the movement, and then exhale to return to the set-up position.

Repetitions: 5 to 8

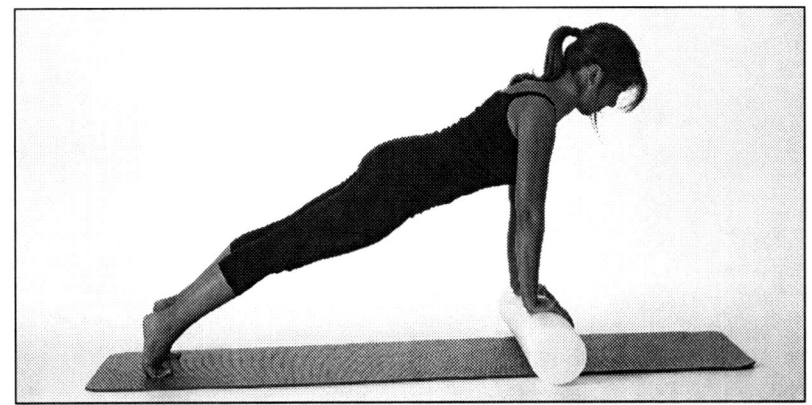
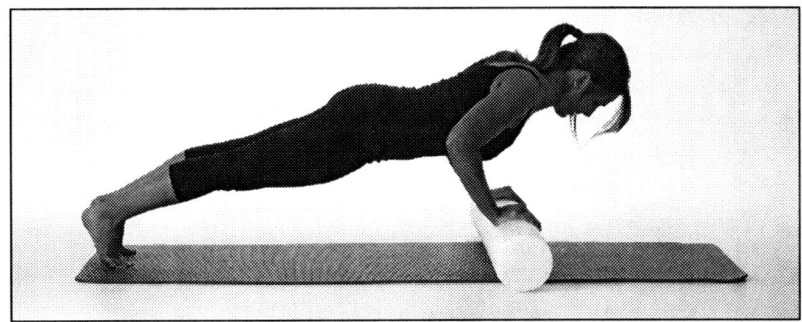
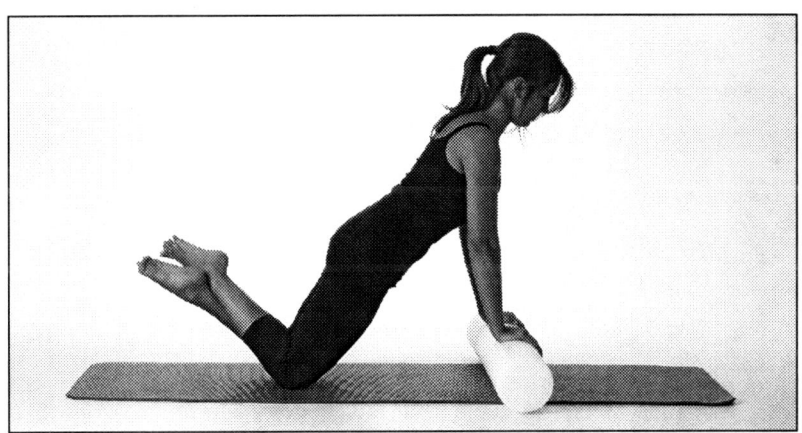
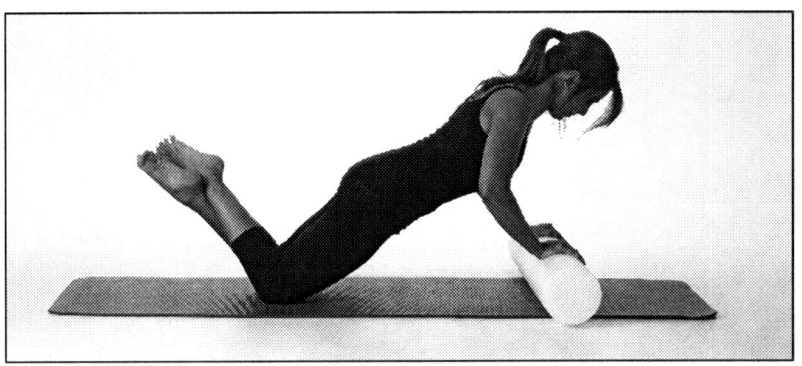

Cat on the Roller

Category: Core and upper-body strengthening

Benefits: This exercise will strengthen the muscles of the arms, chest, and back, and it will improve the stability of the core.

Set-Up: Kneel with your knees directly under your ischial tuberosities and your pelvis in line with the wall in front of you. Position the roller horizontally in front of you.

Movement: Begin rounding forward as if you were rolling off a wall. Try to maintain your hips over your knees throughout the entire exercise. When you are able to reach the roller, place both hands on it, and begin to roll it away from you. Keep your shoulder blades down as you roll all of the way out, bringing your arms over your head and your spine into extension. Return to the start position by posteriorly tilting the pelvis and rounding the spine one vertebra at a time. Remember to keep the hips over the knees so that you challenge your core.

Cues:

- Reach long through the crown of your head.
- Keep your knees over your hips through the entire movement.
- Touch the roller lightly, and do not lean all of your weight into your arms.
- Hold your weight up with your core.
- Place your arms wide on the roller.

Breathing: Inhale to prepare, and exhale as you lower toward the floor. Inhale as you pause at the bottom of the movement, and then exhale to return to the set-up position.

Repetitions: 5 to 8

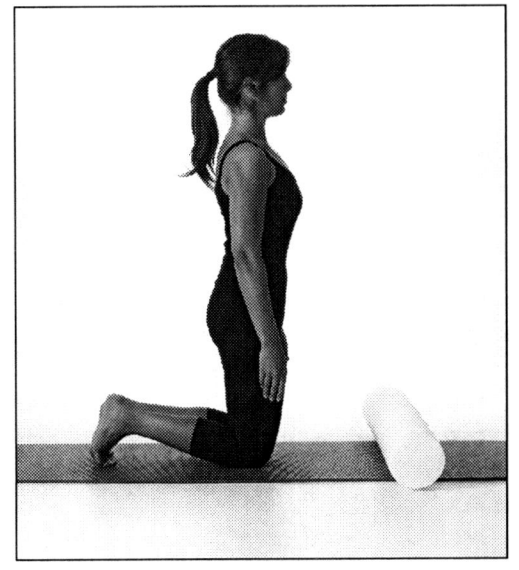
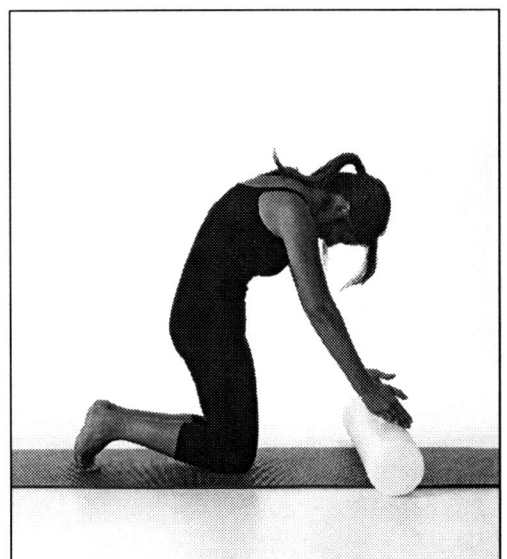
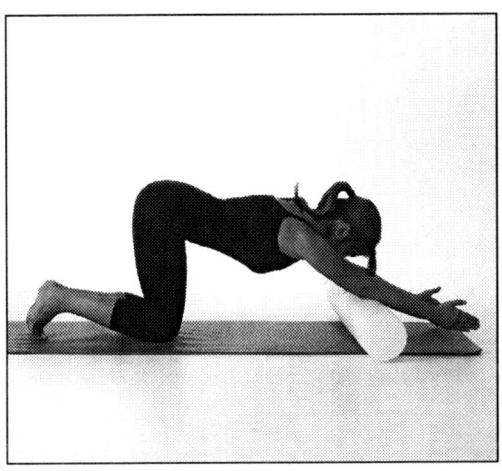
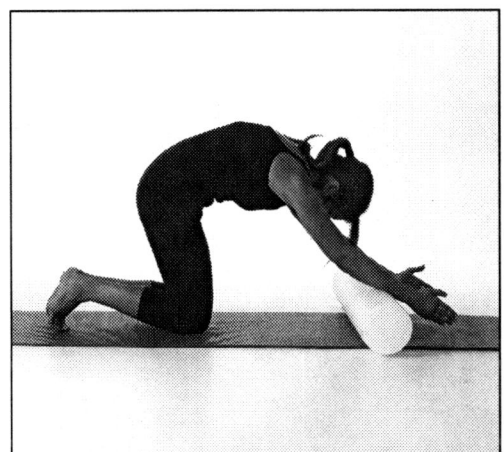

Push-Up With Knees on the Roller

Category: Core and upper-body strengthening

Benefits: This exercise will strengthen the muscles of the arms, chest, and back, and it will improve the stability of the core.

Set-Up: Place your knees on the roller hip-width apart and your hands on the floor with your thumbs and fingers pointing forward. Align your hands directly beneath your shoulders. Position your spine in neutral alignment with the hips extended into a modified plank position.

Movement: While maintaining neutral alignment, bring your upper body toward the floor by bending your elbows. Pause at the bottom of the movement and then return to the set-up position. Continue for the desired repetitions.

Cues:

- Reach long through the crown of your head.
- Keep your back wide and chest open.
- Keep your spine in neutral.

Breathing: Inhale to prepare, and exhale as you lower toward the floor. Inhale as you pause at the bottom of the movement, and then exhale to return to the set-up position.

Repetitions: 5 to 8

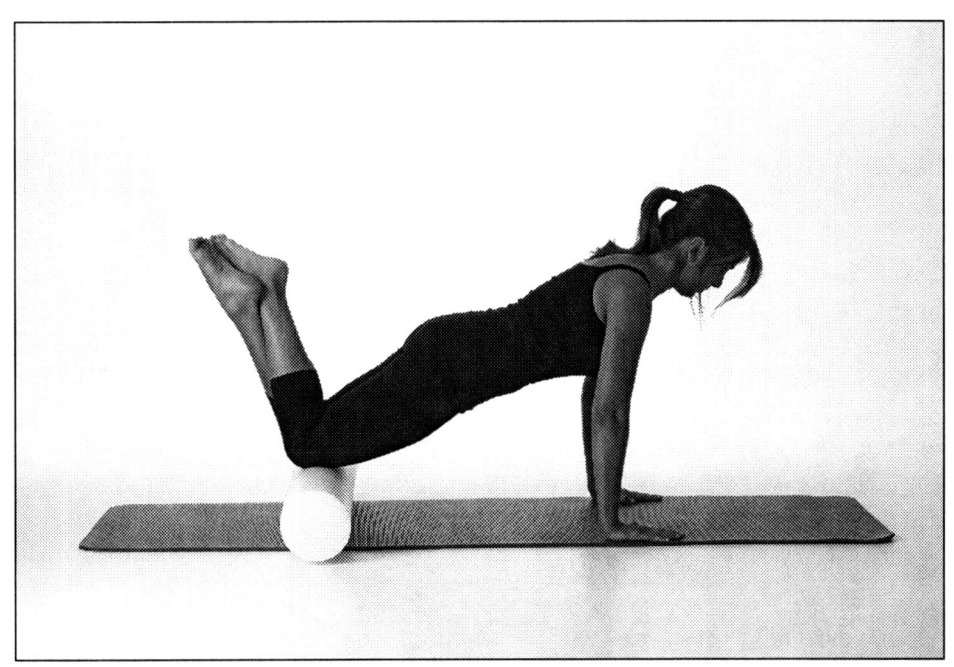
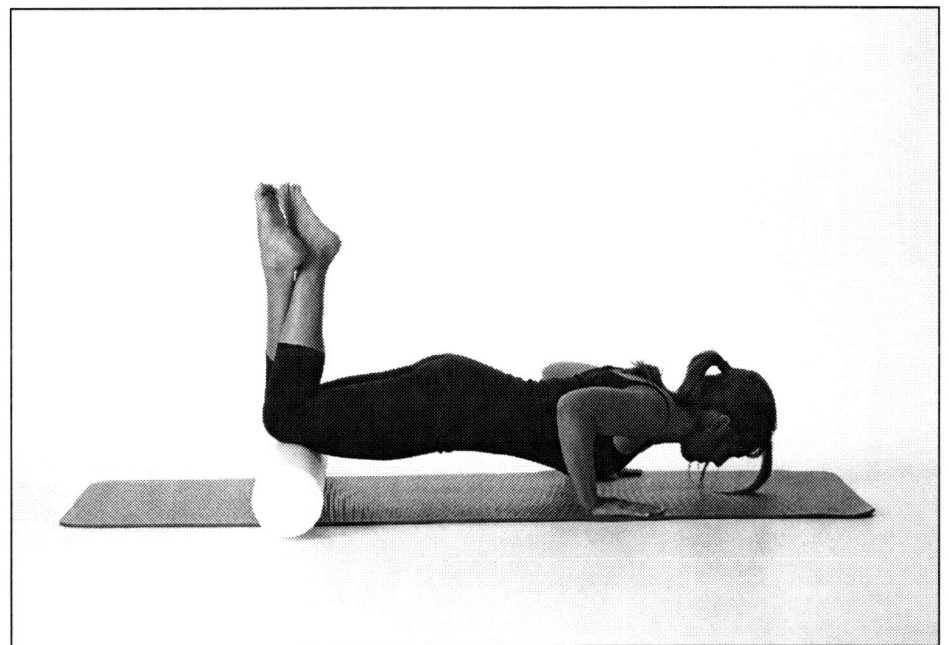

Reverse Plank on Two Rollers

Category: Core and lower-body strengthening; upper-body flexibility and strengthening

Benefits: This exercise will strengthen the core, triceps, chest, and hip extensors. It will also open the chest and shoulders.

Set-Up: Place one roller behind you with your hands on top and your thumbs and fingers facing forward. Position the second roller at your feet.

Movement: Perform a dip to lift your torso onto the roller behind you, and place each calf on the second roller. Zip and wrap your thighs together, and posteriorly tilt your pelvis to lift into a plank position. Hold this position for a few seconds before lowering back to the roller behind you. After you are seated on the back roller, do a dip to lower your torso to the floor.

Cues:

- Open your chest, and keep your shoulders down.
- Do not allow your head to fall back.
- Avoid hyperextension of your elbows.
- Transition back to the roller before returning to the floor to protect your shoulders.

Modifications:

- If you are unable to lift into a reverse plank with the legs fully extended, try the tabletop position. It should be noted that this position will require more flexibility in the upper body.
- If you are a beginning participant, you may need to eliminate the roller beneath your feet.

Progression: With both legs extended, reach one leg at a time toward the ceiling without losing neutral alignment.

Breathing: Inhale to prepare, and exhale as you lift your torso upward. Inhale as you pause at the top, and then exhale as you descend.

Repetitions: 5 to 8

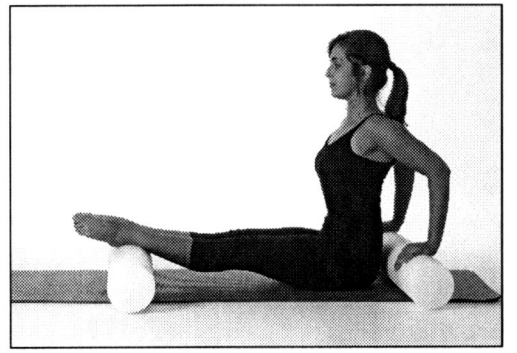 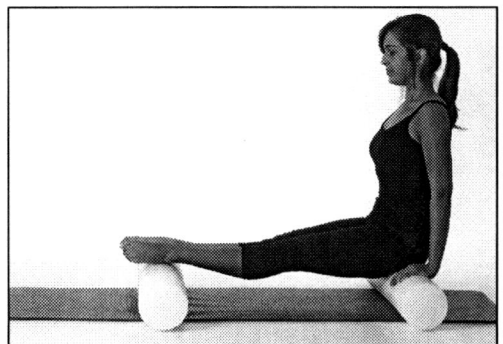
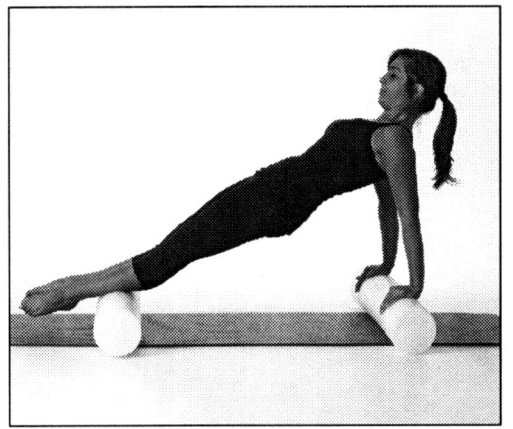 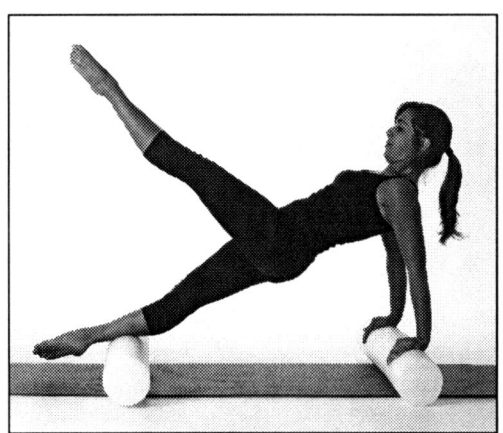
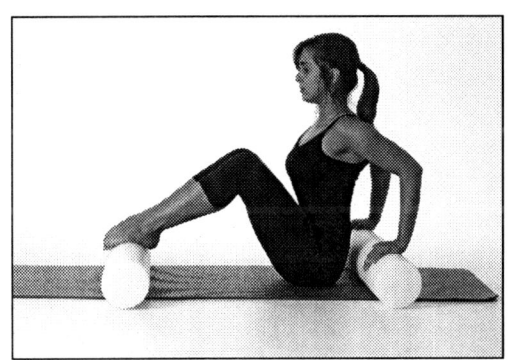 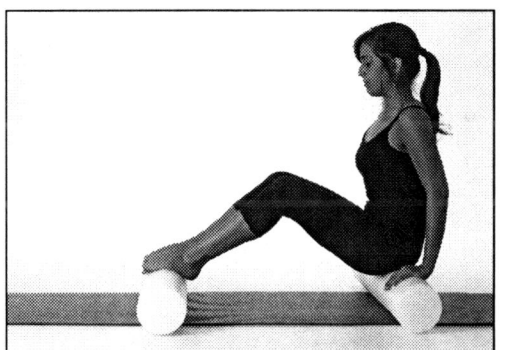
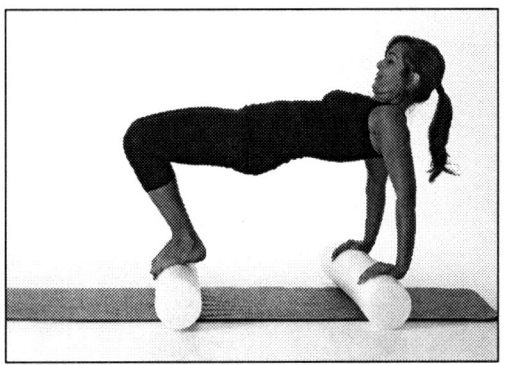

Frog

Category: Lower-body and core strengthening

Benefits: This exercise will strengthen the gluteals and the pelvic floor while lengthening the iliotibial band.

Set-Up: Lie with your back on the mat and your pelvis posteriorly tilted on the foam roller. Place the ring between your ankles with your knees bent toward your chest. Externally rotate your thighs, and maintain lumbar flexion.

Movement: Extend both legs out at an angle in which you can still maintain flexion in the lumbar spine. As you extend your legs, avoid compressing the ring. Just hold it gently so that you use the pelvic floor more than the hip adductors. Maintain the Pilates "V" position with your feet and legs, and then draw your knees back toward your chest.

Cues:

- Keep your knees and second toes aligned.
- Feel a wrapping sensation in your buttocks as you extend your legs.
- Reach your fingers toward your feet to draw your shoulders down your back.

Progression: Use a weighted Pilates ring.

Breathing: Inhale to begin, and exhale as you extend your legs. Inhale and pause at the top, and then exhale to return.

Repetitions: 5 to 8

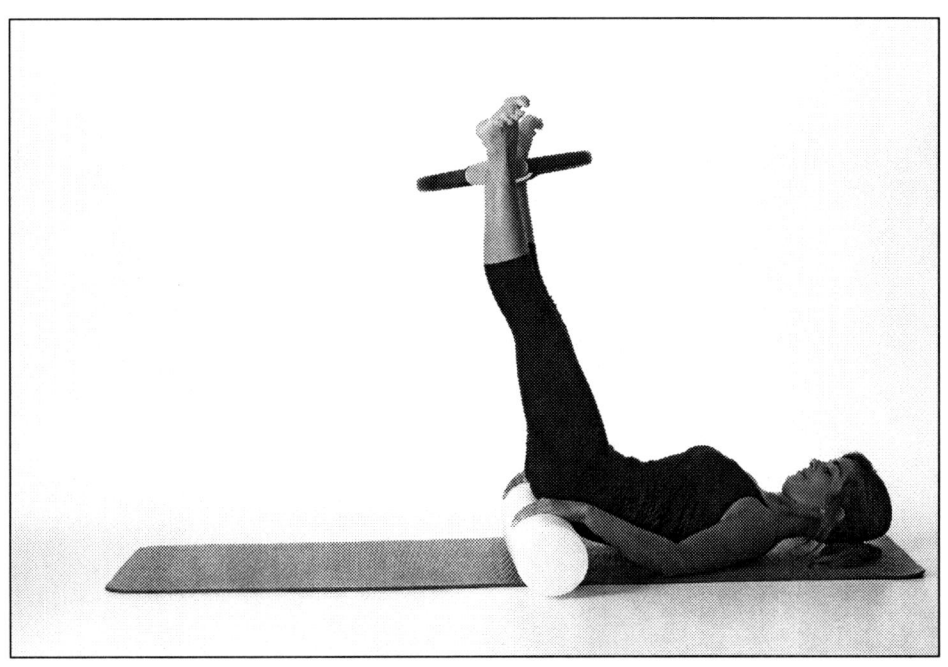
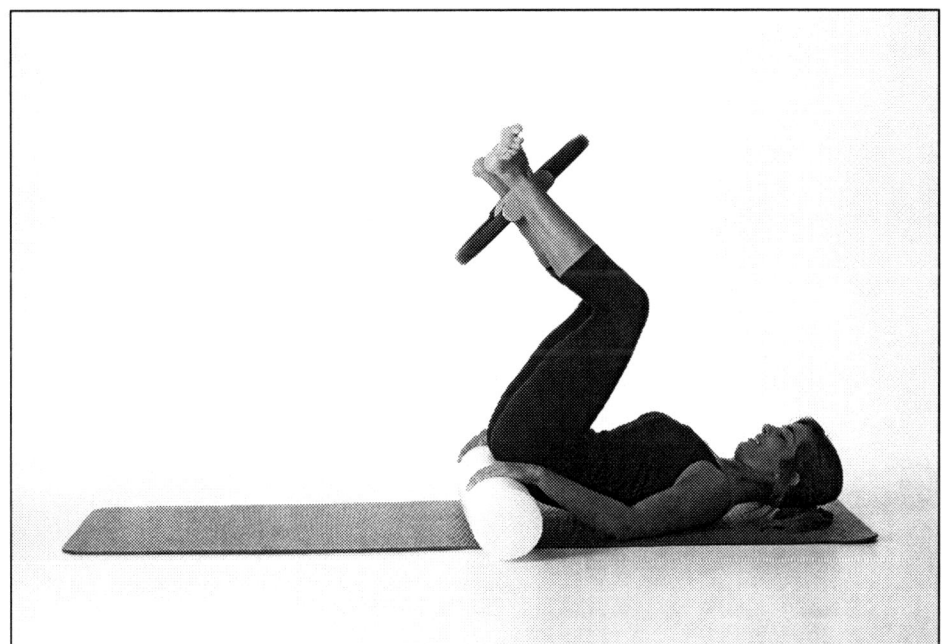

3

The Pilates Ring

Hundred

Category: Warm-up; core strengthening; lumbar flexibility

Benefits: This exercise warms up the body by increasing circulation. It will strengthen the core muscles and increase spinal flexibility.

Set-Up: Lie on your back with your feet hip-width apart and your spine and pelvis in neutral. Place the ring between your legs just above your knees in the tabletop position.

Movement: While maintaining neutral pelvis, curl your head and shoulders off the mat. Reach your arms along your sides, and move them up and down as if you were slapping water. Compress the ring as you exhale for a five count, and release the ring for a five count.

Cues:

- Keep your torso still as the arms move.
- Reach long through the crown of your head.
- Draw your navel to your spine as you exhale.

Modification: If you are unable to maintain the neutral pelvis position, keep your feet on the floor.

Progression: To advance the exercise, place the ring between your ankles, and extend your legs out to a level in which they can maintain neutral pelvis.

Breathing: Inhale for a count of five and exhale for a count of five. Repeat for 10 sets.

Repetitions: 30 to 100 (3 sets of 10; 10 sets of 10)

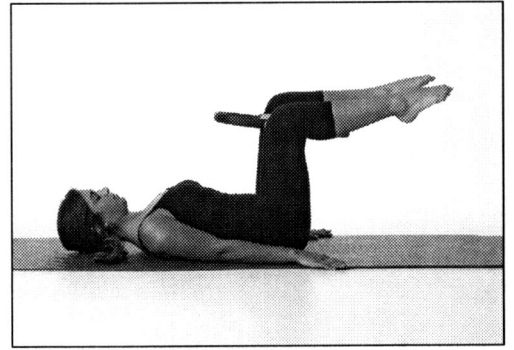 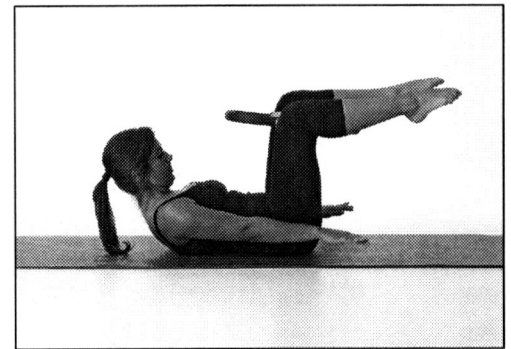

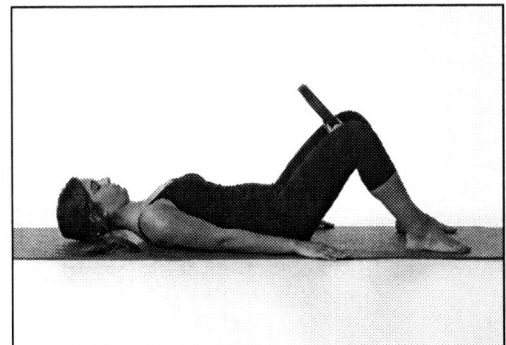 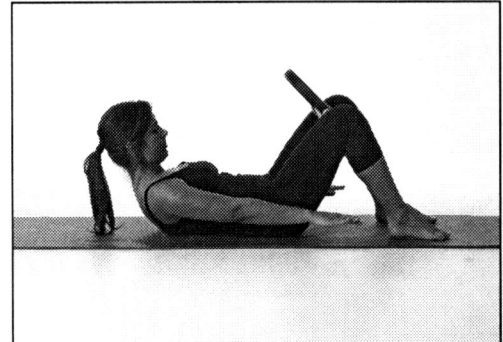

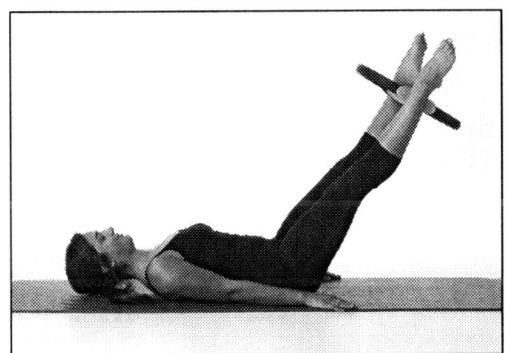 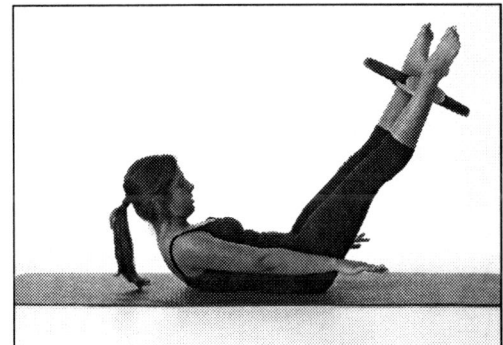

Articulating Bridge

Category: Core strengthening; spinal flexibility

Benefits: This exercise will strengthen the core muscles, gluteal muscles, hamstrings, hip adductors, and pelvic floor. It will also promote flexibility of the spine.

Set-Up: Lie on your back in a hook-lying position with your second toes in line with your kneecaps and your pelvis in neutral. Place the ring above your knees and your arms at your sides.

Movement: Begin the movement by tilting your tailbone toward the ceiling, and then peel one vertebra at a time from the floor. Continue until your hips are fully extended and your ribcage is in line with your pelvis.

Cues:

- Reach your fingers toward your feet as you perform the movement.
- Keep your feet facing forward and your weight to the inside of your foot.

Variation: Perform a straight bridge by maintaining a neutral spine position while moving. Vary the position of the ring to include between the ankles (just above the medial maleolus), above the knee but with the legs inside the circle, and at the ankles with the legs inside the circle.

Progression: Hold in the top position, and squeeze the ring three to five times while breathing.

Breathing: Inhale to begin and exhale as you articulate the spine.

Repetitions: 5 to 8

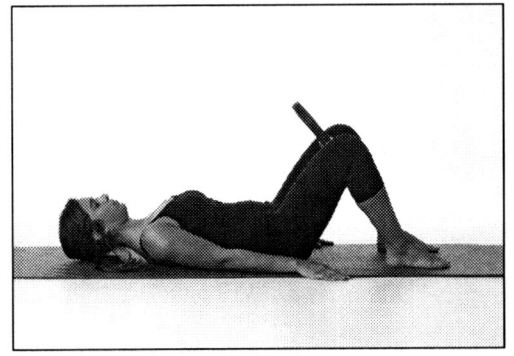
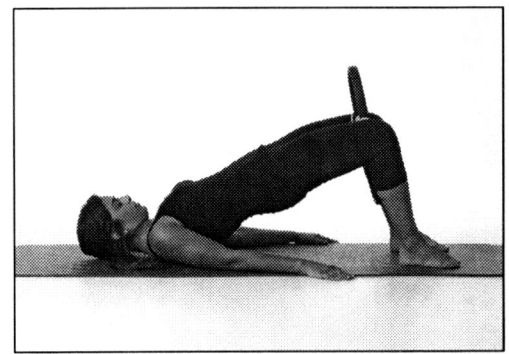
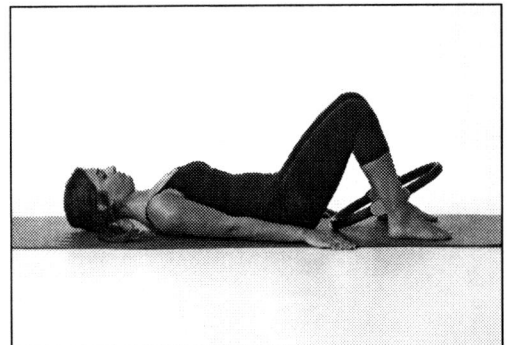
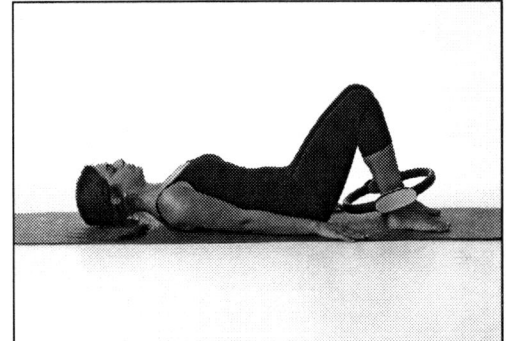
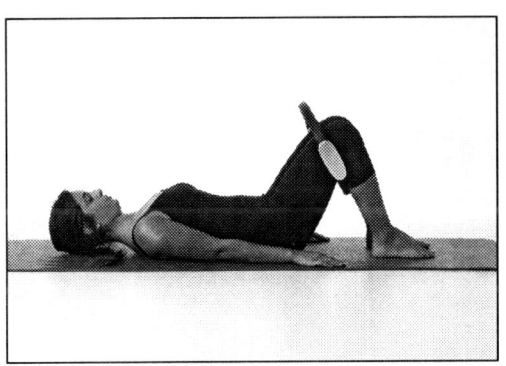
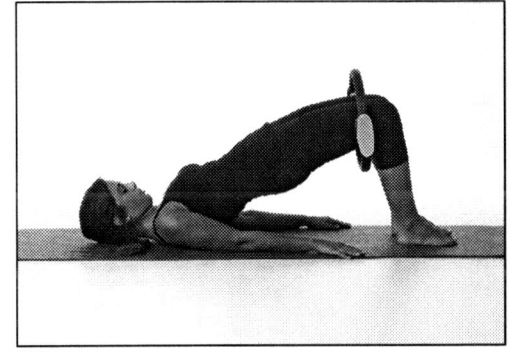

Cervical Nod

Category: Posture training

Benefits: This exercise will teach proper alignment of the head and neck for the stomach series exercise. It is an excellent way to work against the forward-head posture.

Set-Up: Lie on your back in the hook-lying position. Align your heels with your ischial tuberosities and your knees with your second toes. Position your pelvis in neutral, and place the ring under your head. Hold the handle of the ring with your hands with your elbows bent.

Movement: Perform a small cervical nod without taking your head off the ring or the ring off the floor. Continue to roll up into the hundred position, while gently pulling with your arms. Keep the back of your head on the ring throughout the movement. Roll up only to where you can keep your pelvis in neutral and then return to the set-up position.

Cues:

- Keep a long neck, and do not let your chin touch your chest.
- Think of lifting your head with your upper abdomen.

Breathing: Inhale to begin, and exhale as you roll up. Inhale at the top, and exhale as you roll down.

Repetitions: 5 to 8

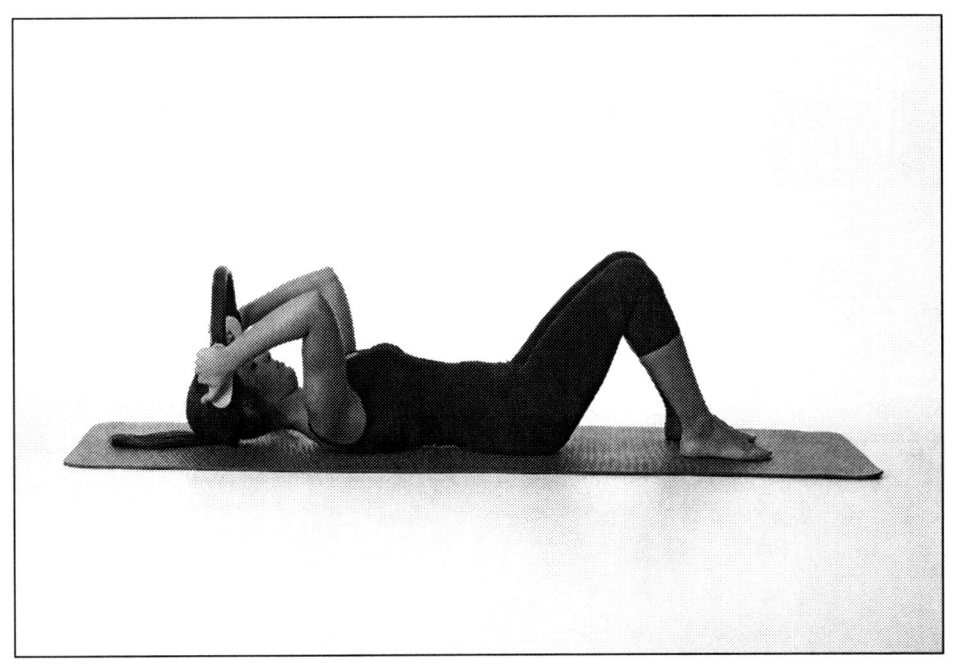

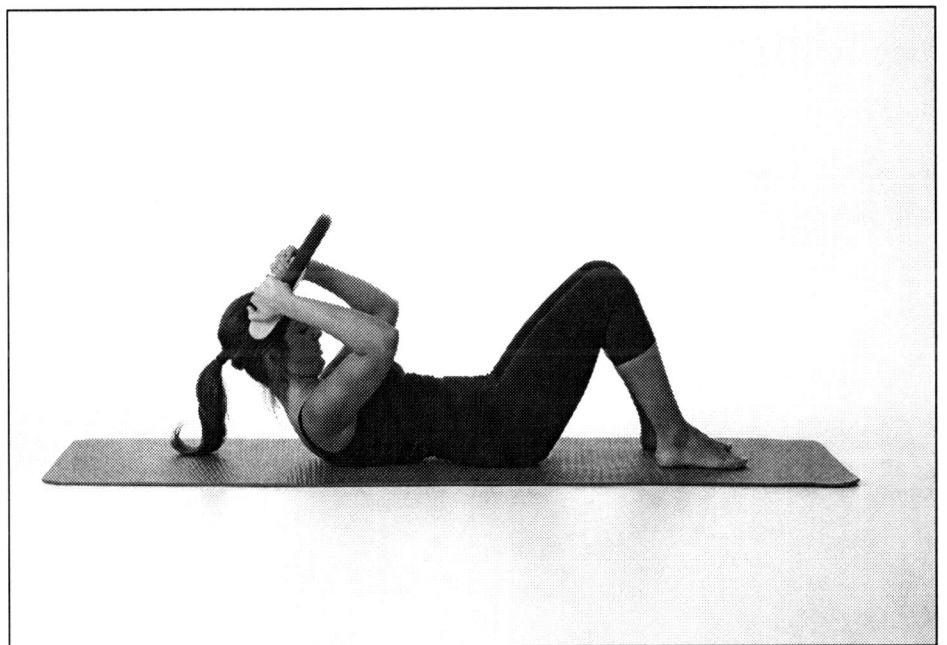

Roll-Up

Category: Core strengthening and spinal flexibility

Benefits: This exercise will strengthen the core muscles and promote flexibility of the spine.

Set-Up: Lie on your back with one ring in your hands and one ring between your heels. Maintain the ring position at the feet by outwardly rotating your hips in the Pilates "V" position.

Movement: Begin the movement by raising your arms over your head without lifting your ribcage. Perform a cervical nod as you roll up one vertebra at a time. At the top, round your spine forward over your legs into a "C" curve. Keep your shoulders down, and look through the ring as you roll back. Repeat for the desired repetitions.

Cues:

- Look through the ring like a camera when it is in your hands.
- Zip and wrap the legs around the ring to engage the pelvic floor.
- Keep a long neck, and do not let your chin touch your chest.

Progression: Use a weighted Pilates ring.

Breathing: Inhale to begin, and exhale as you roll up. Inhale at the top, and exhale as you roll down.

Repetitions: 5 to 8

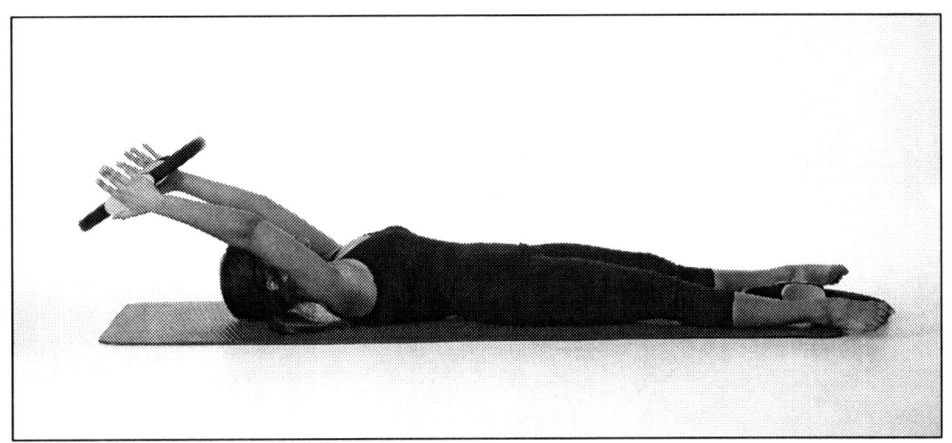

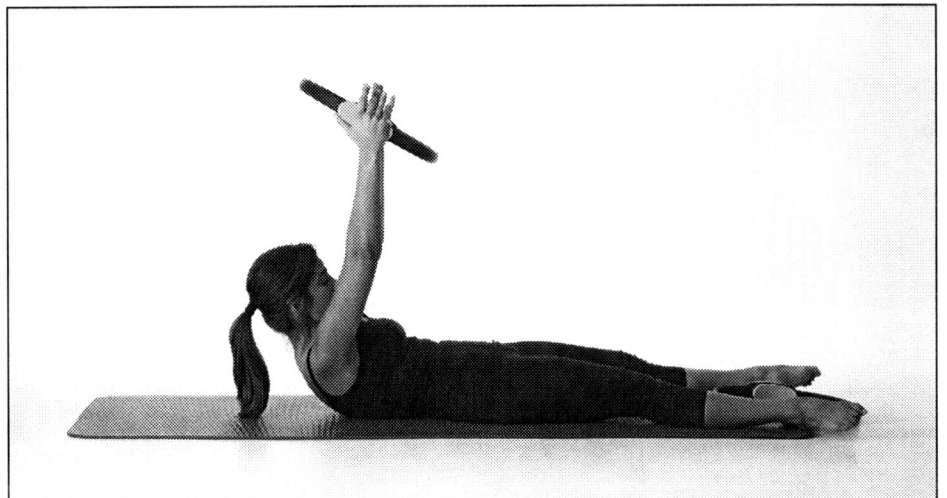

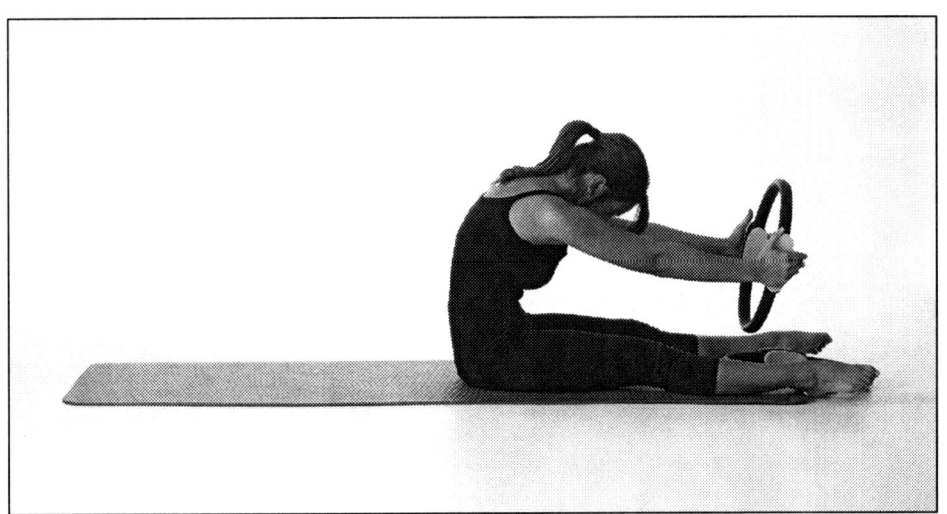

Hip Adductor

Category: Lower-body strengthening and flexibility; core strengthening and stability

Benefits: This exercise will strengthen the hip adductor and abductor muscles while lengthening the iliotibial band. Maintaining the neutral alignment will also challenge core stability.

Set-Up: Lie in side-lying neutral alignment with your bottom leg inside the ring and your top leg resting on the handle of the ring. For side-lying neutral, line your back up with the mat and place your legs slightly in front of you. Stack your hips and shoulders, and reach your top leg long to line up your pelvis in the transverse plane. The ring will lean slightly away from you as you reach your top leg long. Rest your head on your lower arm, and use the top arm for balance.

Movement: While in neutral alignment, compress the ring by adducting the upper leg. Then, relax the top leg, and reach the bottom leg into adduction.

Cues:

- Keep your hips stacked.
- Keep your shoulders down stacked and open.
- Reach long out of your legs.
- Maintain alignment of the ASIS of the pelvis.

Progression: Lift your upper body off the floor to rest onto your forearm.

Variation: Attempt to retrace the inside circle of the ring with your bottom leg. Repeat in the opposite direction.

Breathing: Inhale to begin, and exhale on the movement.

Repetitions: 5 to 8 on each side

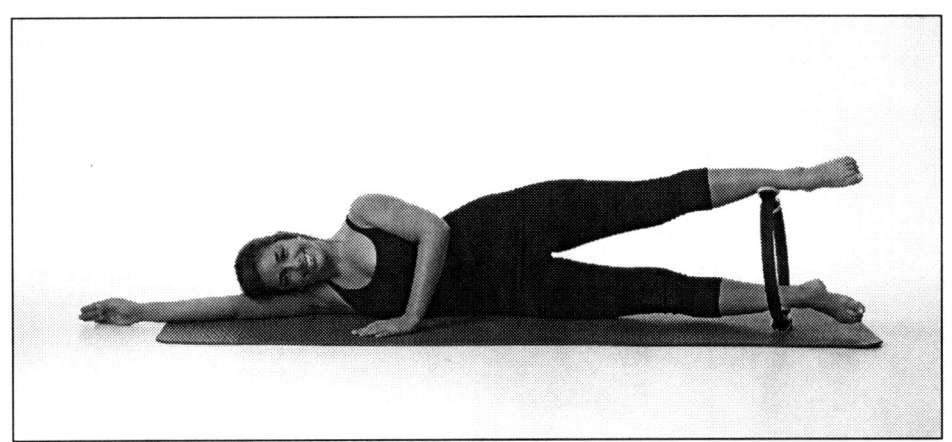
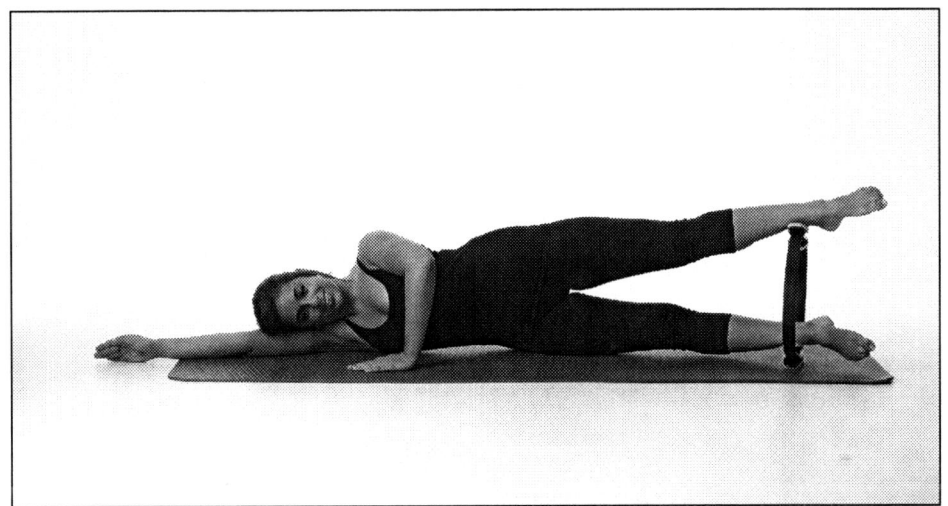
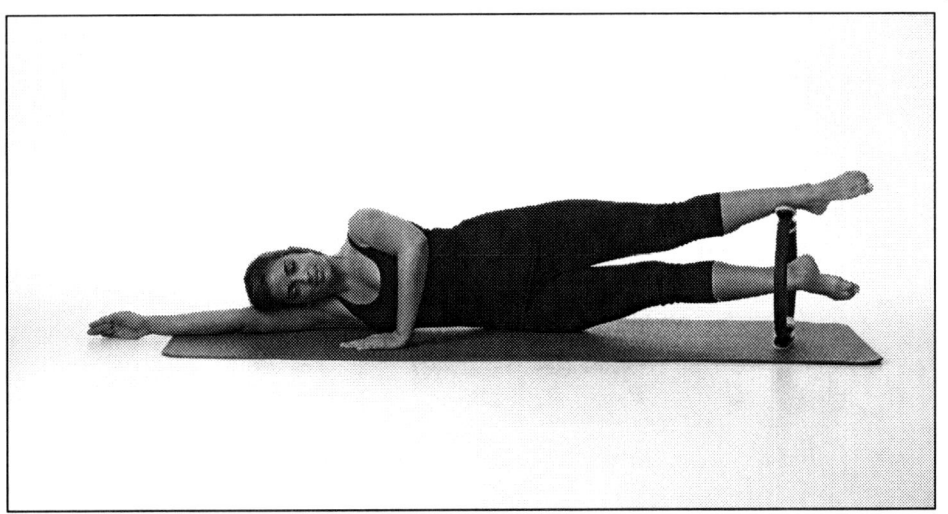

Shoulder Stability

Category: Upper-core stability

Benefits: This exercise will improve stability of the shoulder girdle.

Set-Up: Lie in side-lying neutral alignment. Place the ring in front of you with your hand positioned on the top handle.

Movement: While maintaining this neutral position, compress the circle with 10 pounds of force.

Cues:

- Keep your hips stacked during the movement.
- Keep your shoulders down your back as you compress the ring.
- Reach long through the crown of your head to lengthen your neck.

Modification: Bend the bottom leg to create a larger base of support.

Variation: Reposition the ring in all ranges of shoulder movement, and also try in a seated position.

Breathing: Inhale to prepare, and exhale as you press into the ring.

Repetitions: 5 to 8 on each side

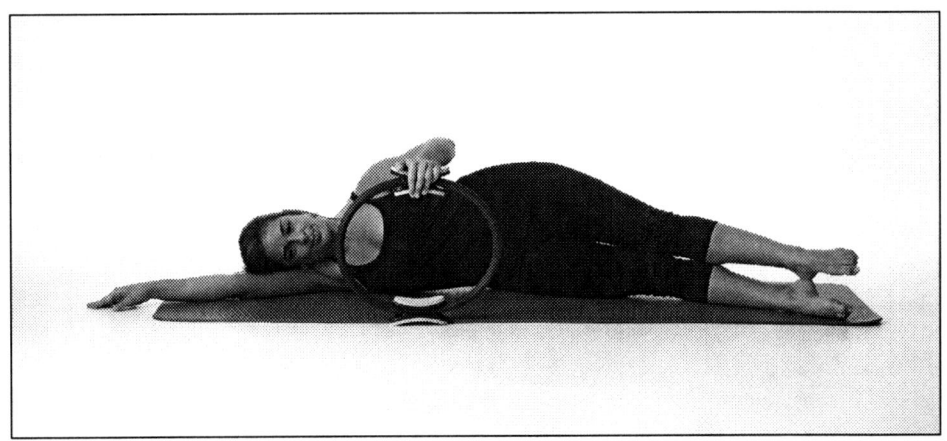
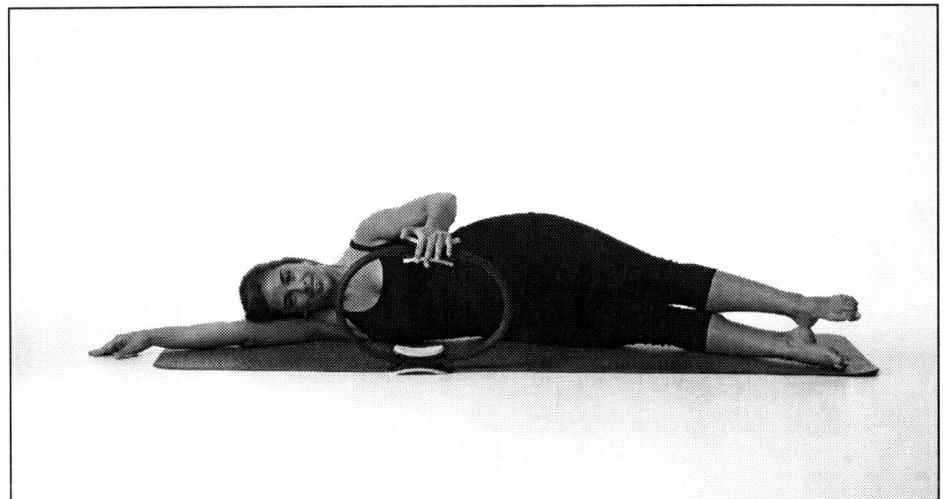
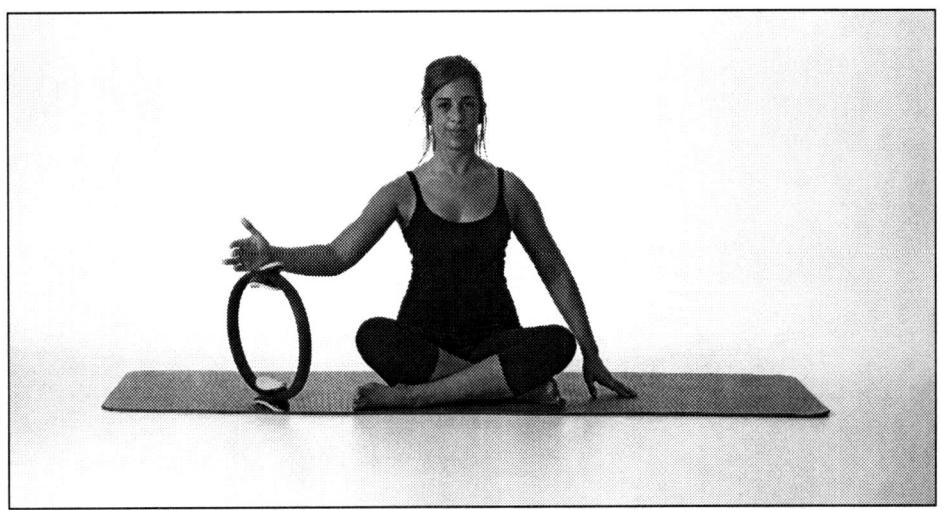

Shave the Head

Category: Upper-body strengthening

Benefits: This exercise will strengthen the shoulders and upper back.

Set-Up: Sit with your legs in a bowl position. The soles of your feet will be touching, and your knees are flexed.

Movement: Hinge forward at the hips with a flat back. Place both hands on the pads of the ring, and bring the ring behind your head. Extend your arms out from your head. Return your arms while pressing lightly into the ring. Continue for the desired repetitions.

Cues:

- Reach through the crown of the head.
- Keep your chest open and shoulders down.
- Stay flexed at the hips.

Modifications:

- If you are unable to bring your hands behind your head, place the ring in front of your forehead.
- If you cannot hinge without a flat back, try sitting on box.

Breathing: Inhale as your arms extend, and exhale as they return.

Repetitions: 5 to 8

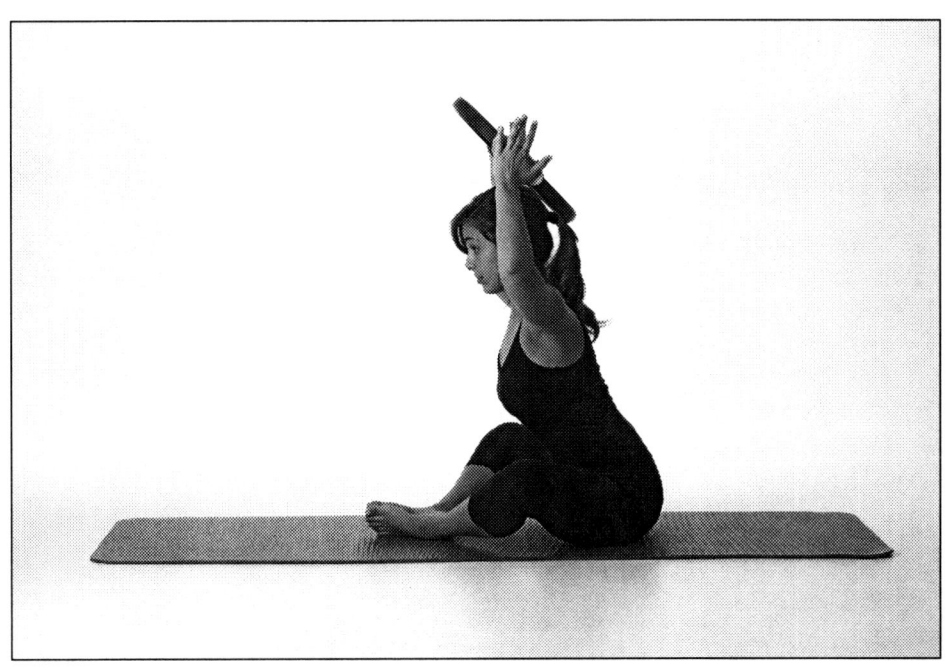
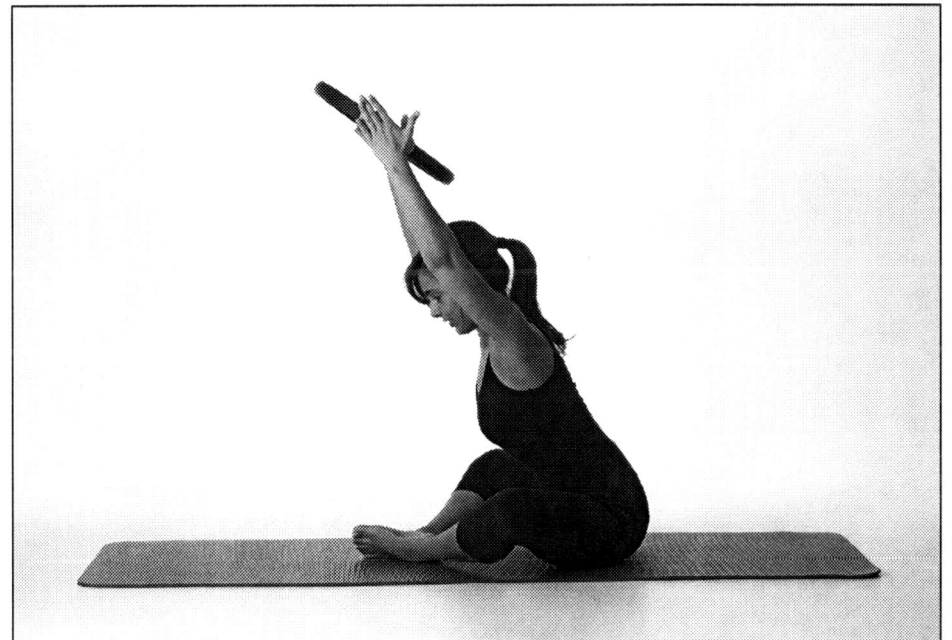

Spine Stretch

Category: Flexibility of the spine and lower extremities

Benefits: This exercise will lengthen the hamstrings and paraspinal muscles.

Set-Up: Sit in a neutral seated position with your legs as wide as your pelvis. Place the ring on the floor between your legs balanced on one pad. Place both hands on the top pad with the elbows soft and shoulders down.

Movement: Begin by nodding your chin and then round your spine up and over. Imagine that you are rounding over a ball on your lap. The ring will compress as the spine moves. Avoid movement at the shoulder.

Cues:

- Stay lifted tall on the ischial tuberosities (sitting bones) as you perform the movement.
- Keep your shoulders down your back with a slight bend at the elbow.

Modifications: Use an alternate seated position if neutral pelvis cannot be achieved in a long sit position. The best choice is to sit on a small box or wedge.

Breathing: Inhale to prepare, and exhale as you compress the ring.

Repetitions: 5 to 8

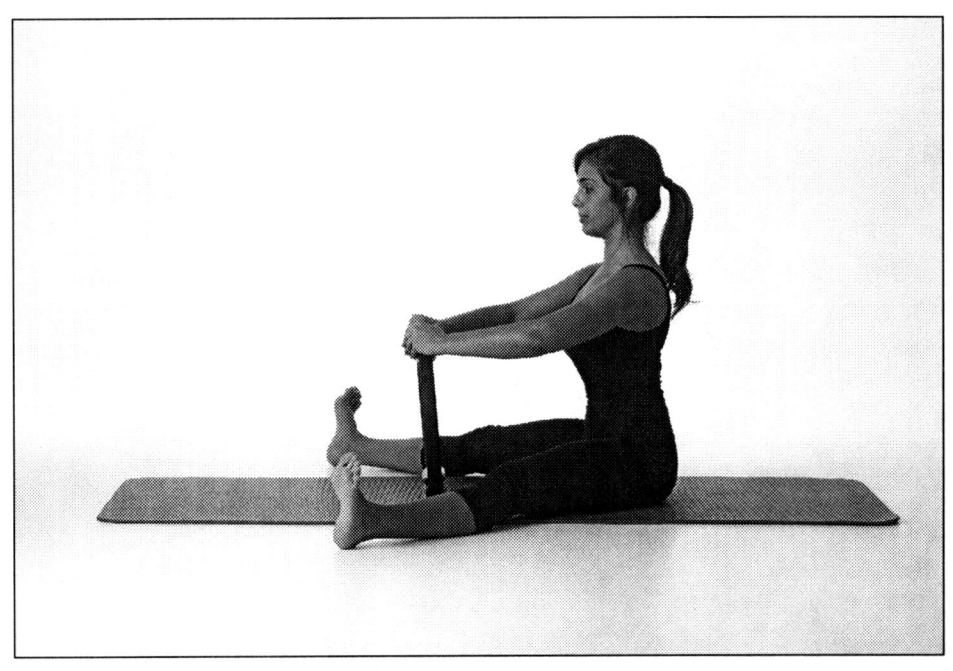
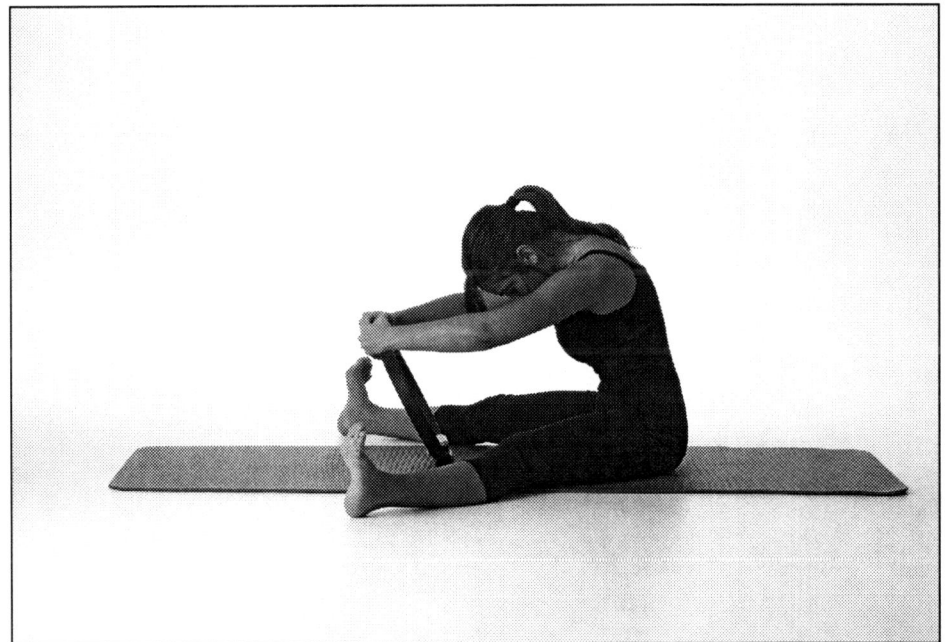

Mermaid

Category: Spine and hip flexibility

Benefits: This exercise will lengthen the quadratus lumborum and hip muscles. It also will strengthen the quadratus lumborum and the abdominal obliques.

Set-Up: Sit mermaid-style with one hip internally rotated and the other hip externally rotated. Reach your ischial tuberosities to the floor, and align your pelvis and ribcage with the wall in front of you. Place the ring slightly in front of you on the side of the front leg with your hand on the top handle.

Movement: Round your spine in a "C" curve to the side compressing the ring. Keep your shoulder stable, and compress the ring with your torso.

Cues:

- Keep your torso square with the wall in front of you as you move.
- Lift your spine up and away from the floor without lifting your pelvis.
- Keep your shoulders down as your compress the ring.

Modifications: If you are unable to sit in mermaid position, sit on a small box.

Variation: While rounded to the side toward the ring, rotate the spine and place the other hand on the pad of the ring. Stay rotated, and extend into a flat-back position. The ring will lean toward you as you extend the spine.

Breathing: Inhale to prepare, and exhale as you round your spine toward the ring. For the swan variation, you can inhale as the spine extends to help lengthen the spine.

Repetitions: 5 to 8 on each side

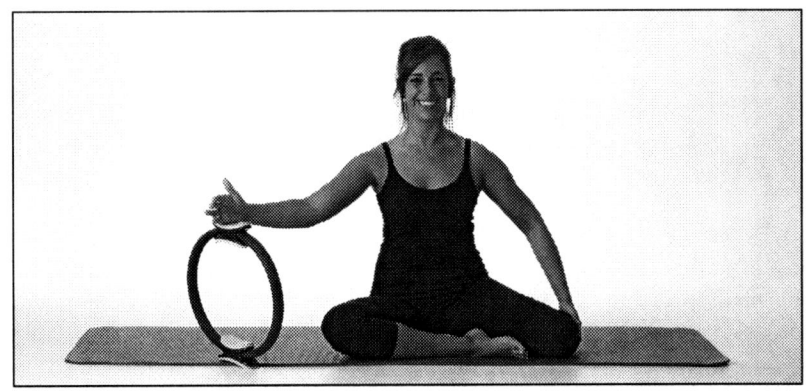
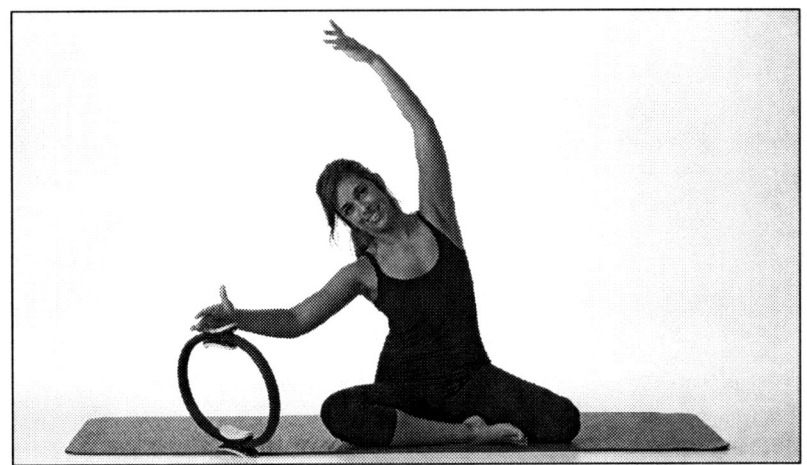
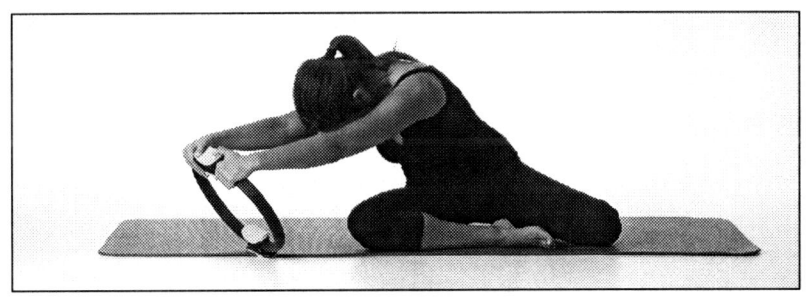
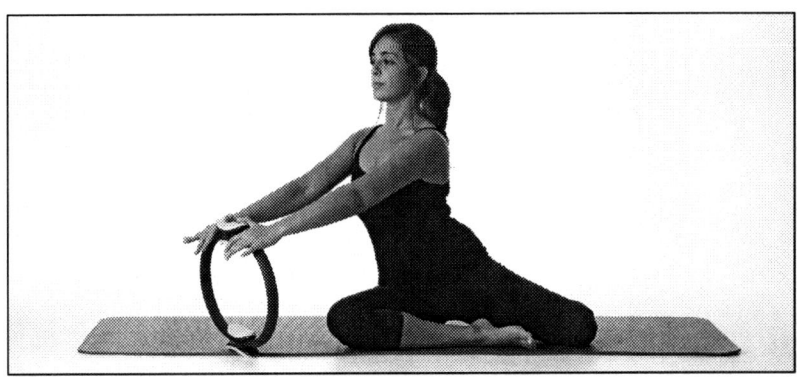

Ribcage Arms

Category: Posture training; shoulder stability

Benefits: This exercise will teach scapulohumeral rhythm and increase shoulder range of motion.

Set-Up: Stand in the Pilates "V" posture, and hold the ring in your hands. Outwardly rotate your shoulders, and slightly bend your elbows. Align your ASIS with your pubic bone so that your pelvis is in the frontal plane. Stack your ribcage on top of your pelvis aligning the 10th rib with your ASIS. Square your shoulders and hips with the wall in front of you.

Movement: While maintaining the standing alignment, raise the ring as high as you can without elevating your shoulder girdle. When you begin to lose alignment or raise your shoulder girdle, return to the start position and begin again. Continue for the desired repetitions.

Cues:

- Reach long through the crown of your head.
- Be sure to keep the ring in the shape of a circle. If it compresses into an egg shape, you are using your chest and bicep muscles.

Modification: Perform this exercise in the hook-lying supine position.

Breathing: Inhale as you raise the ring, and exhale as you bring it back to the starting position.

Repetitions: 5 to 8

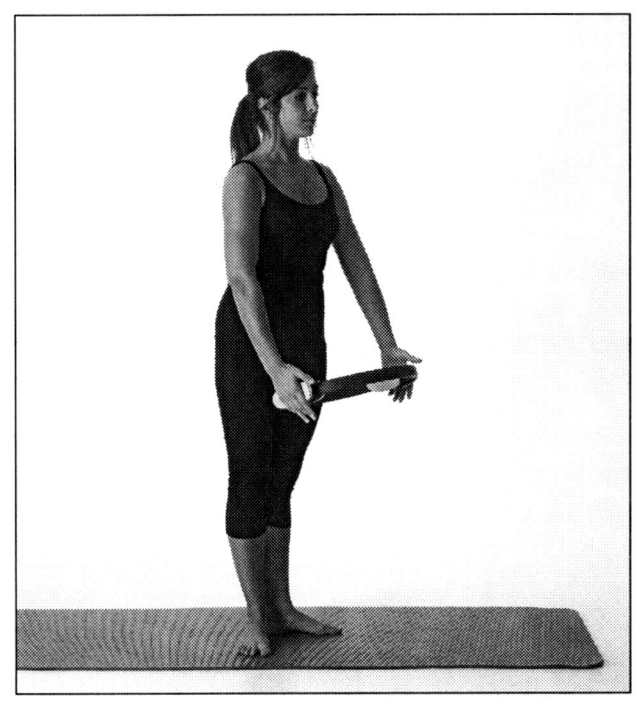
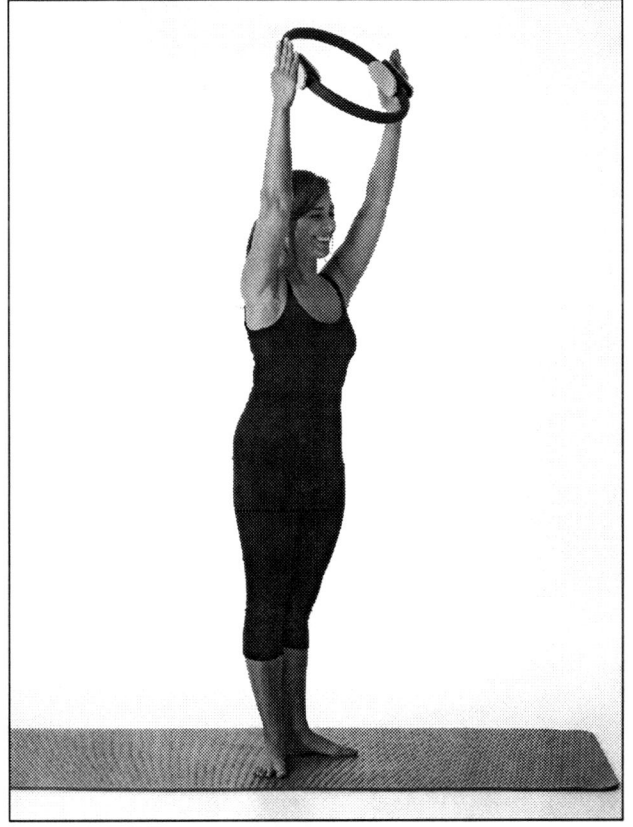

Pliés and Footwork

Category: Lower-body strengthening and flexibility; posture training

Benefits: This exercise will strengthen the muscles of the legs and pelvis. It is also a fantastic teaching tool for standing posture.

Set-Up: Stand in the Pilates "V" position, and place the ring between your ankles just above the medial maleolus. Align your ASIS with your pubic bone so that your pelvis is in the frontal plane. Stack your ribcage on top of your pelvis aligning the 10th rib with your ASIS. Square your shoulders and hips with the wall in front of you.

Movement: In the Pilates "V" position, perform a plié, keeping your spine in neutral alignment. Maintain the plié as you raise onto your toes, and then return to the starting position. Perform this combination for the desired repetitions and then repeat in the other direction.

Cues:

- Keep your tailbone between your legs as you perform the pliés.
- Reach long through the crown of your head.
- Keep your knees and second toes aligned during the pliés.
- Be sure to keep the ring in the shape of a circle. If it compresses into an egg shape, you are using your adductors too much.

Breathing: Use a breath with each movement.

Repetitions: 5 to 8

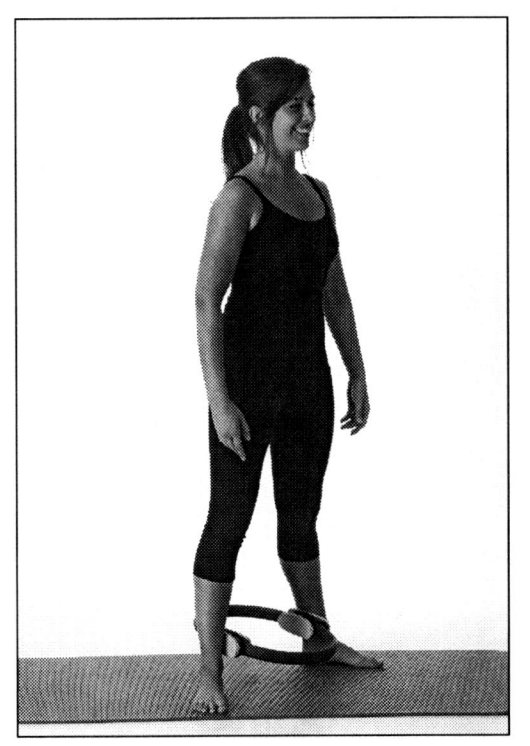
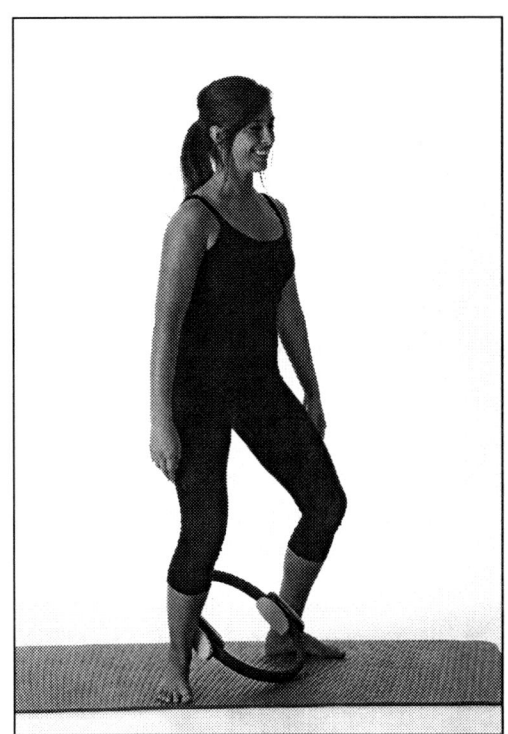
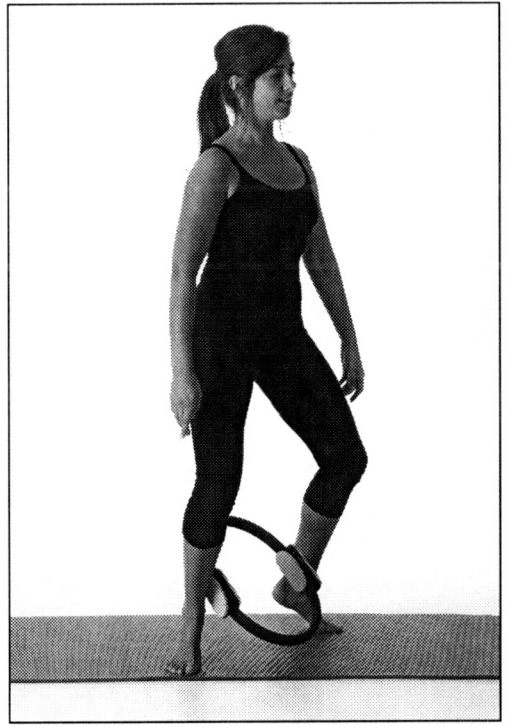
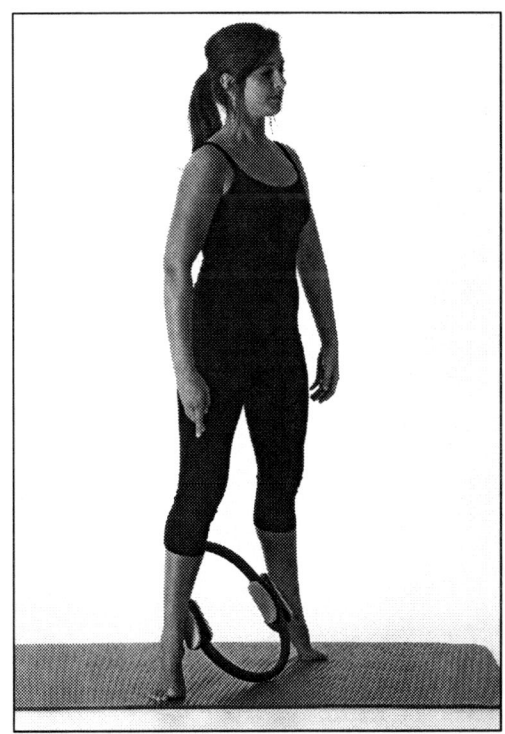

Squats

Category: Lower-body strengthening; posture training

Benefits: This exercise will strengthen the muscles of the legs and work against medial collapse at the knee.

Set-Up: Sit in a chair or on the sitting box with your legs inside the ring and your knees in line with your second toes. The ring should be placed just above your knee, and you should open gently into it.

Movement: Lean forward from the hips as you shift your weight forward to come to stand. Maintain the position of the ring above your knees as you come to a complete standing position. Return to the sitting position without losing the ring position. Repeat for the desired repetitions.

Cues:

- Be sure to lean forward to come to a stand. Think: "Nose over toes."
- Return to the seated position with the same thought of "nose over toes."

Modification: If you are unable to maintain the ring position, start from a higher seat. Decrease the seat height as your form improves.

Breathing: Inhale as you move sit to stand, and exhale as you return to the seated position.

Repetitions: 5 to 8

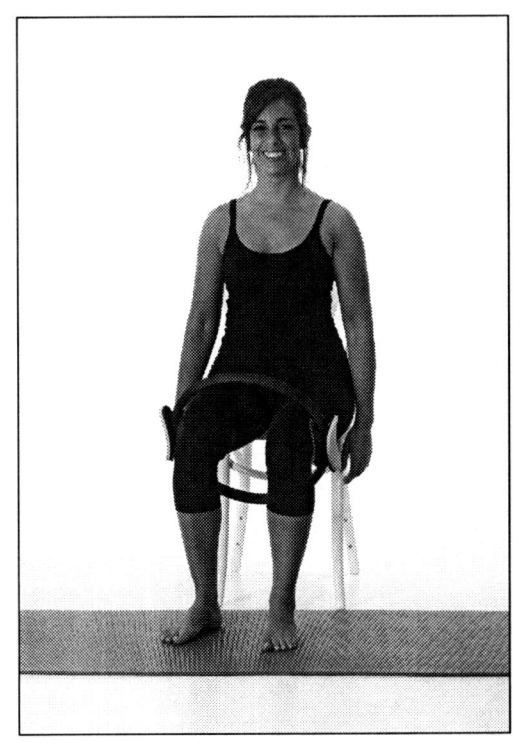
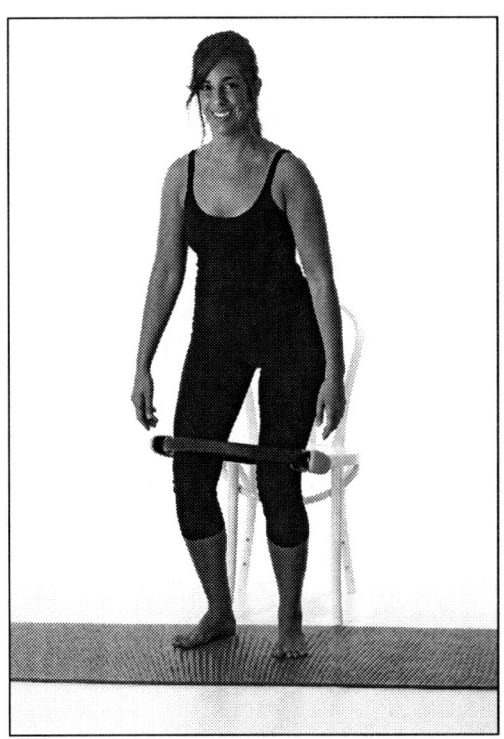
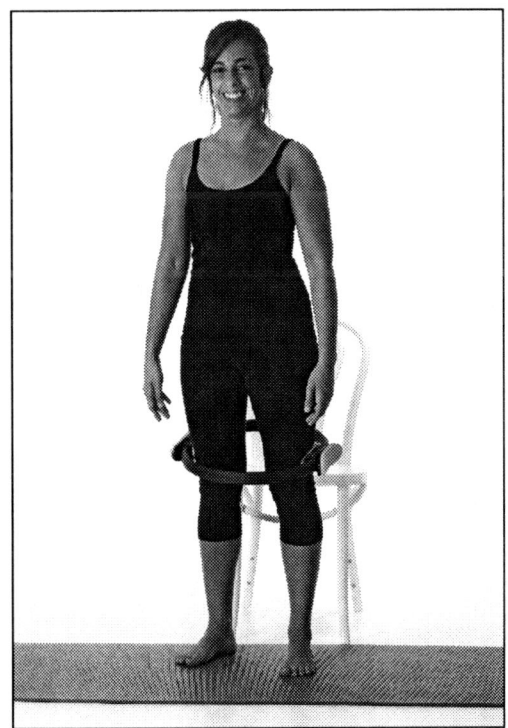

Hamstring Stretch

Category: Lower body and spinal flexibility

Benefits: This exercise will lengthen the muscles of the back and hamstrings and increase the stability of the upper core.

Set-Up: Hold one pad of the ring with both hands. Stand up tall in neutral alignment with your hips in neutral and your feet as wide as your pelvis.

Movement: While holding the ring in front of you, begin rounding your spine one vertebra at a time as if you are rounding away from a wall. Make sure that as you reach toward the floor that you maintain a rounded spine from your hip to the crown of your head. Once you get to the floor, place the other pad of the ring onto the floor. Stay in a rounded spine as you compress the ring five times.

Cues:

- Stay forward on the front of your feet in order to help facilitate the calf and hamstring stretch.
- Keep your shoulders down and back as you round forward.
- Reach through the crown of your head during the movement.

Modifications: If you have short hamstrings and cannot reach all the way to the floor, place the ring on a box or step.

Breathing: Inhale to begin, and exhale as you round forward. Exhale each time that you compress the ring.

Repetitions: 5 to 8

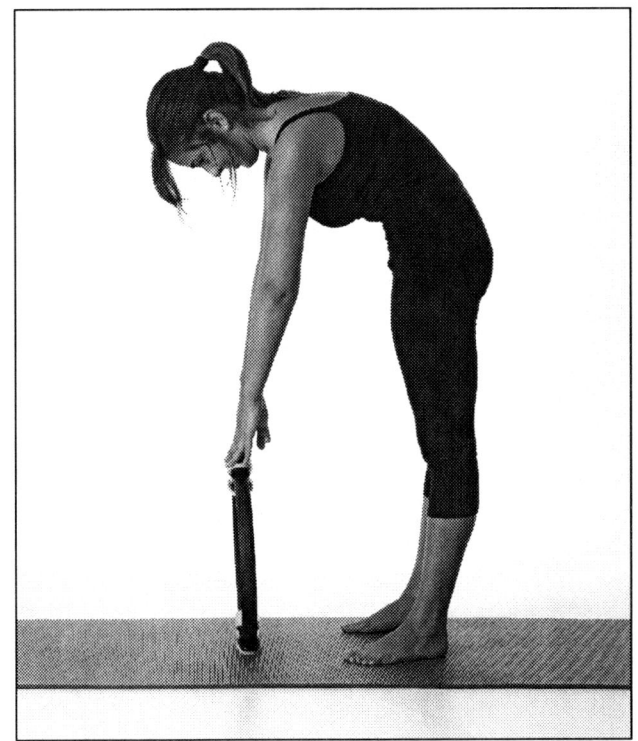

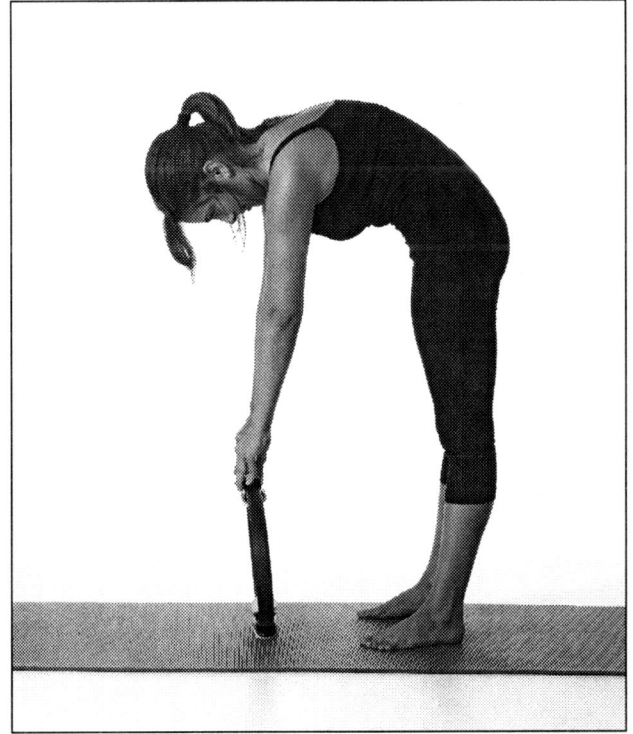

Long Back Stretch

Category: Upper-body flexibility; postural awareness

Benefits: This exercise will lengthen the muscles of the chest, neck, and arms. It will also strengthen the upper back.

Set-Up: Hold the ring behind your back with one hand on each pad. The ring should be parallel to your body. Position your body in Pilates posture with the feet and hips in Pilates "V."

Movement: While holding the ring behind you with the elbows extended, reach your arms behind you without elevating the shoulders or losing the Pilates posture. Repeat this motion for the desired repetitions and then begin the second movement. For the second movement, slide the ring up and down your back by bending the elbows without elevating the shoulders. Be sure to keep the elbows pointed backward. Repeat this motion for the desired repetitions.

Cues:

- Keep the elbows pointed backward.
- Reach through the crown of your head during the movement.

Progression: Tie the two movements together to create a circle, and repeat in each direction for the desired repetitions.

Breathing: Inhale or exhale with each movement.

Repetitions: 5 to 8

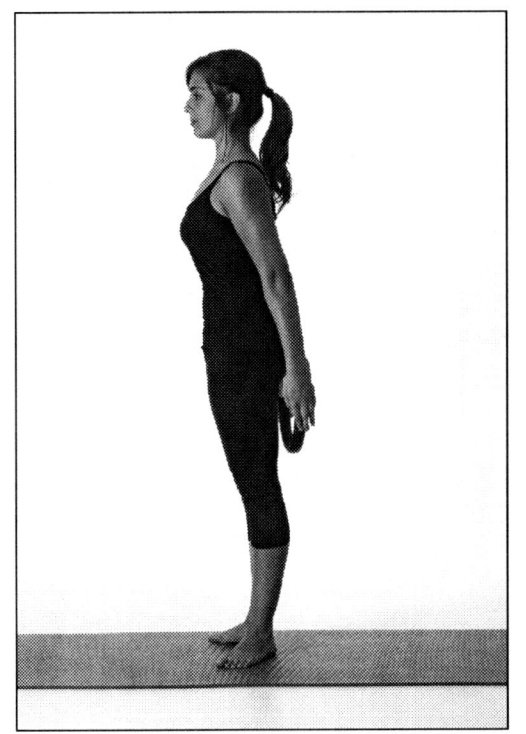
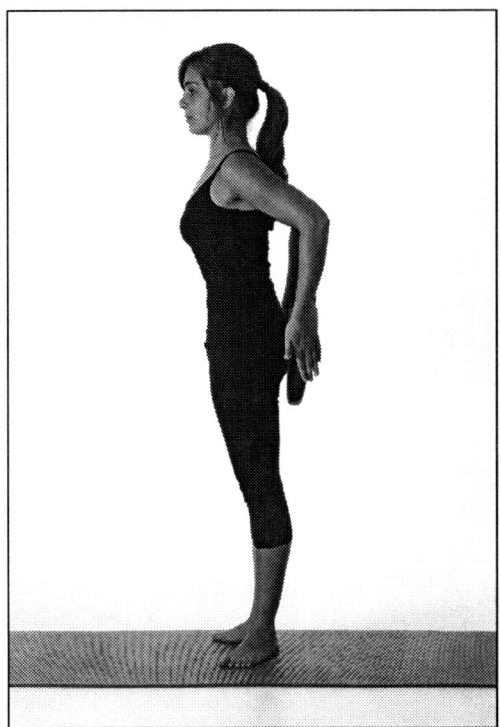
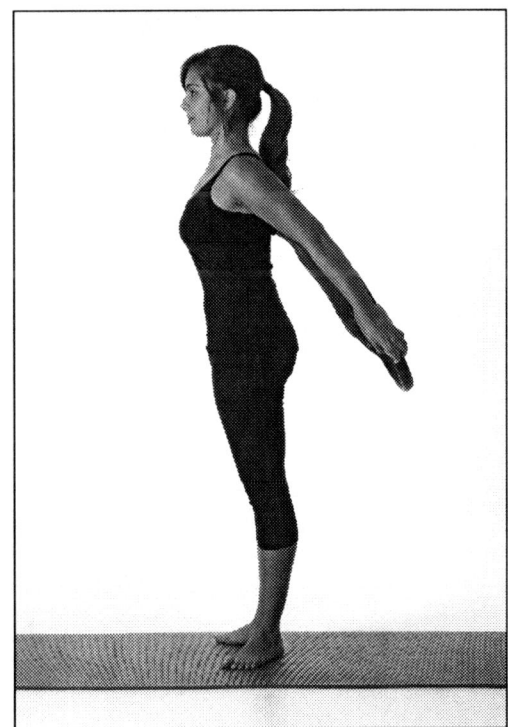

87

Hip Extension/Frog

Category: Hip extensor strengthening

Benefits: This exercise will increase core strength and disassociate hip motion from spine motion.

Set-Up: Lie face down with your pelvis in neutral, hips in external rotation, knees bent, and the ring between your ankles. Lace your fingers together, and place your hands under your forehead. Align your ribcage with your pelvis and draw your navel to your spine.

Movement: Reach your knees away as you gently extend your hips without moving your lumbar spine or your head. Release slowly back to the floor, maintaining the bent knee position. Repeat for the desired repetitions.

Cues:

- Keep your lumbar spine still as the hips move.
- Try not to push down through your head.
- Draw your navel to your spine as you exhale.

Progression: Gently outwardly rotate the hips to squeeze the ring in both the raised and lowered positions.

Breathing: Inhale to prepare, and exhale as you lift.

Repetitions: 5 to 8

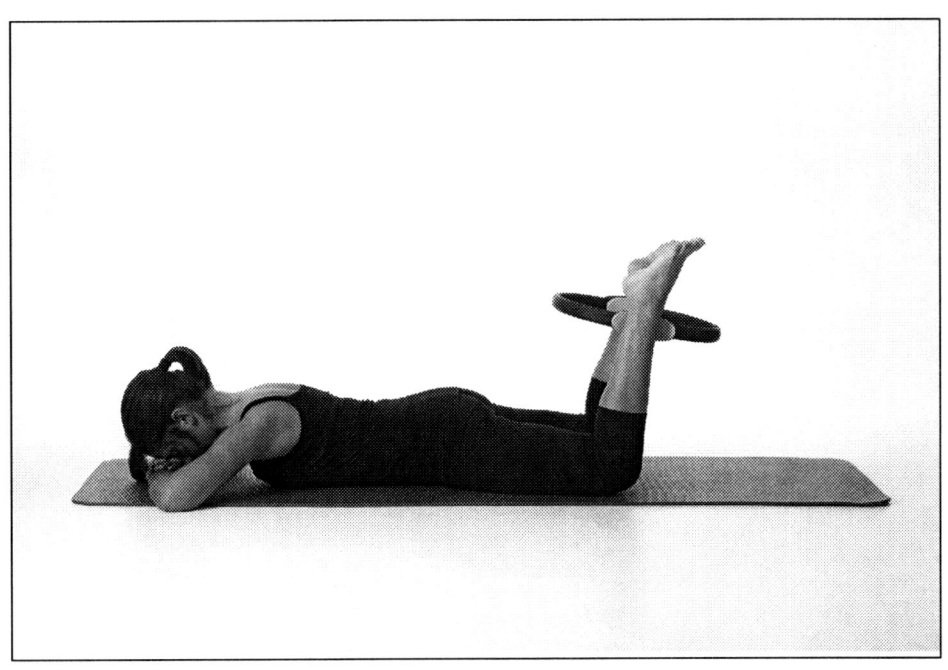

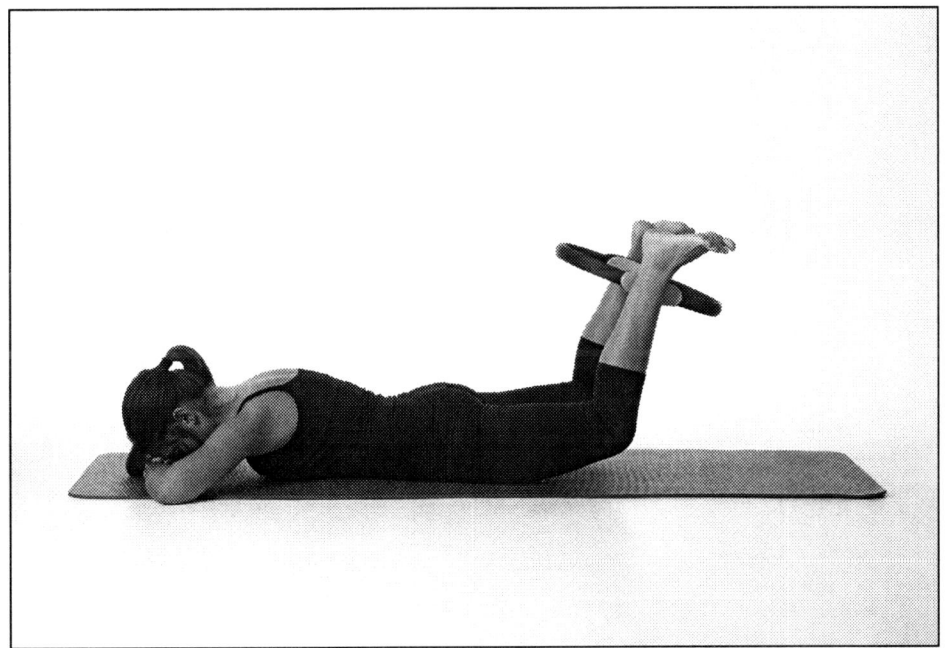

4

The Spine Corrector

Arm Circles

Category: Spinal mobility, especially thoracic and lumbar extension

Benefits: This exercise will improve the stability of the shoulder girdle and the mobility of the thoracic and lumbar spine.

Set-Up: Lie with your upper back against the barrel. Attempt to wrap your lumbar spine over the barrel and perform a cervical nod to reach out of the top back of your head. Extend your legs out long in outward rotation, and bring the back of your sacrum against the curve of the barrel. Your arms should be extended along your sides with your chest open.

Movement: Reach your arms up and overhead while maintaining the position against the barrel. Continue the circle around to return to your sides. Repeat for the desired repetitions, and then reverse the direction. Keep the circle small if you are unable to maintain the set-up position.

Cues:

- Reach long out of the back of your head.
- Draw your ribs into the barrel.
- Keep the bottom of the sacrum against the barrel to maintain lumbar extension and support.

Modification: Make the circles very small with control.

Progression: You may use small weights for this exercise or a weighted bar for just shoulder flexion and extension.

Breathing: Inhale as you reach overhead, and exhale for the remainder of the circle. To perform the opposite direction, inhale as you abduct the arms to the sides, and exhale as you return them to the start position.

Repetitions: 5 to 8

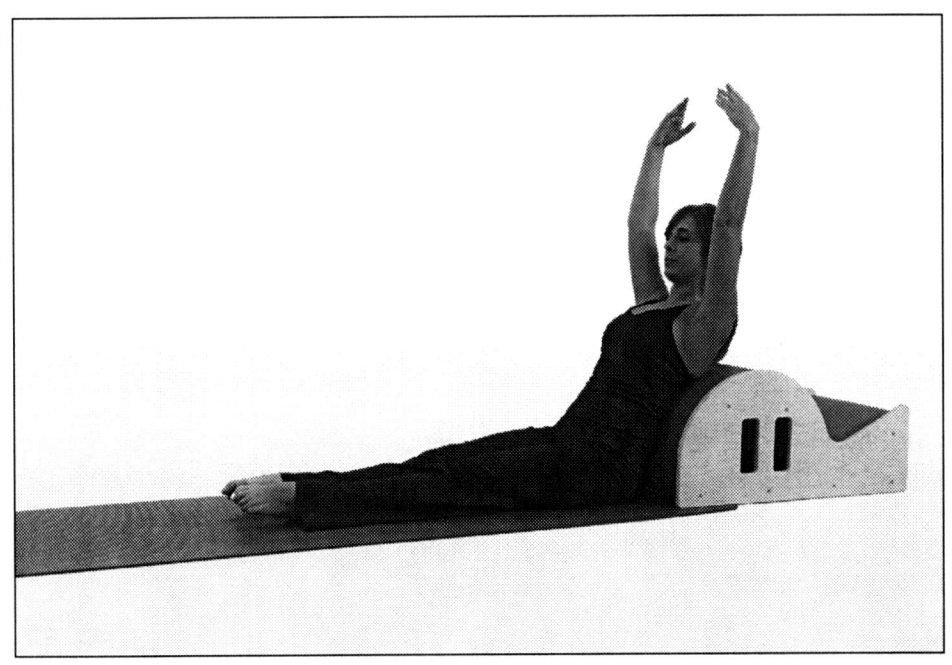

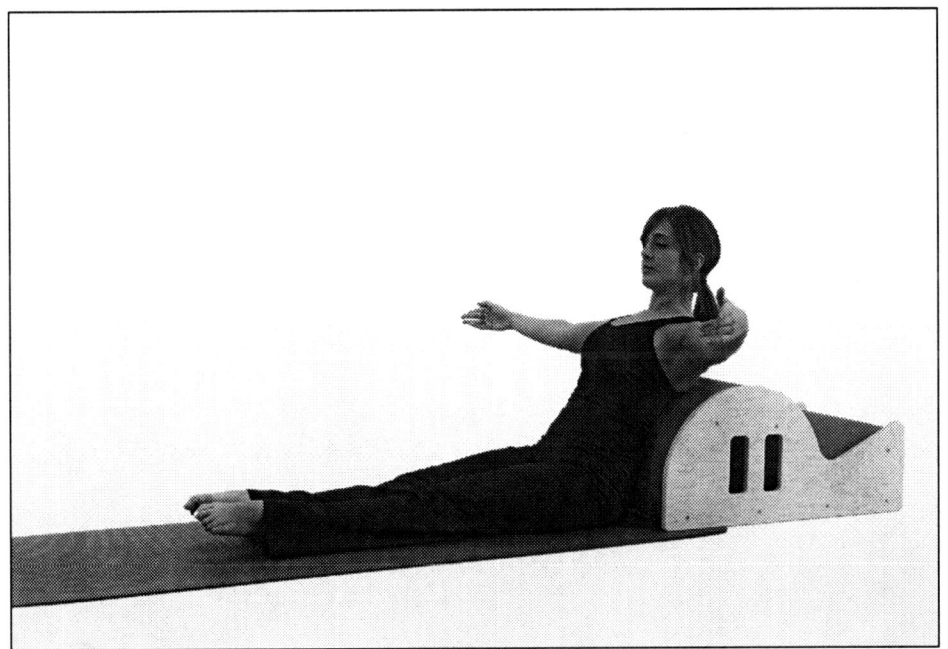

Leg Circles

Category: Hip mobility; disassociation of hip and spinal movement

Benefits: This exercise will improve the mobility of the hips and the stability of the pelvic girdle.

Set-Up: Lie supine with your buttocks against the barrel. Draw the knees to the chest as you pull the barrel under you to support your lower back using the side handles. Hold these handles as you lengthen your neck and extend your legs up in outward rotation. Position the lumbar spine in flexion with the pelvis in a posterior tilt.

Movement: While holding the handles and keeping contact with the barrel for spine support, abduct the legs and begin to circle out. Draw the legs down and together, and then bring them back to the starting position. Repeat the circles for the desired repetitions, and then reverse the direction. The exercise may be done in hip outward rotation or hip neutral. Avoid hip internal rotation.

Cues:

- Reach long out of the leg.
- Relax the neck, and reach long out of the top back of the head.
- Keep the bottom of the sacrum against the barrel to maintain lumbar support.

Modification: Make the circles very small with control.

Breathing: Inhale as you open the legs and draw them down and together. Exhale as you bring the legs up into the starting position. For the opposite motion, inhale as you draw the legs down, and exhale as you abduct and return to the starting position.

Repetitions: 5 to 8

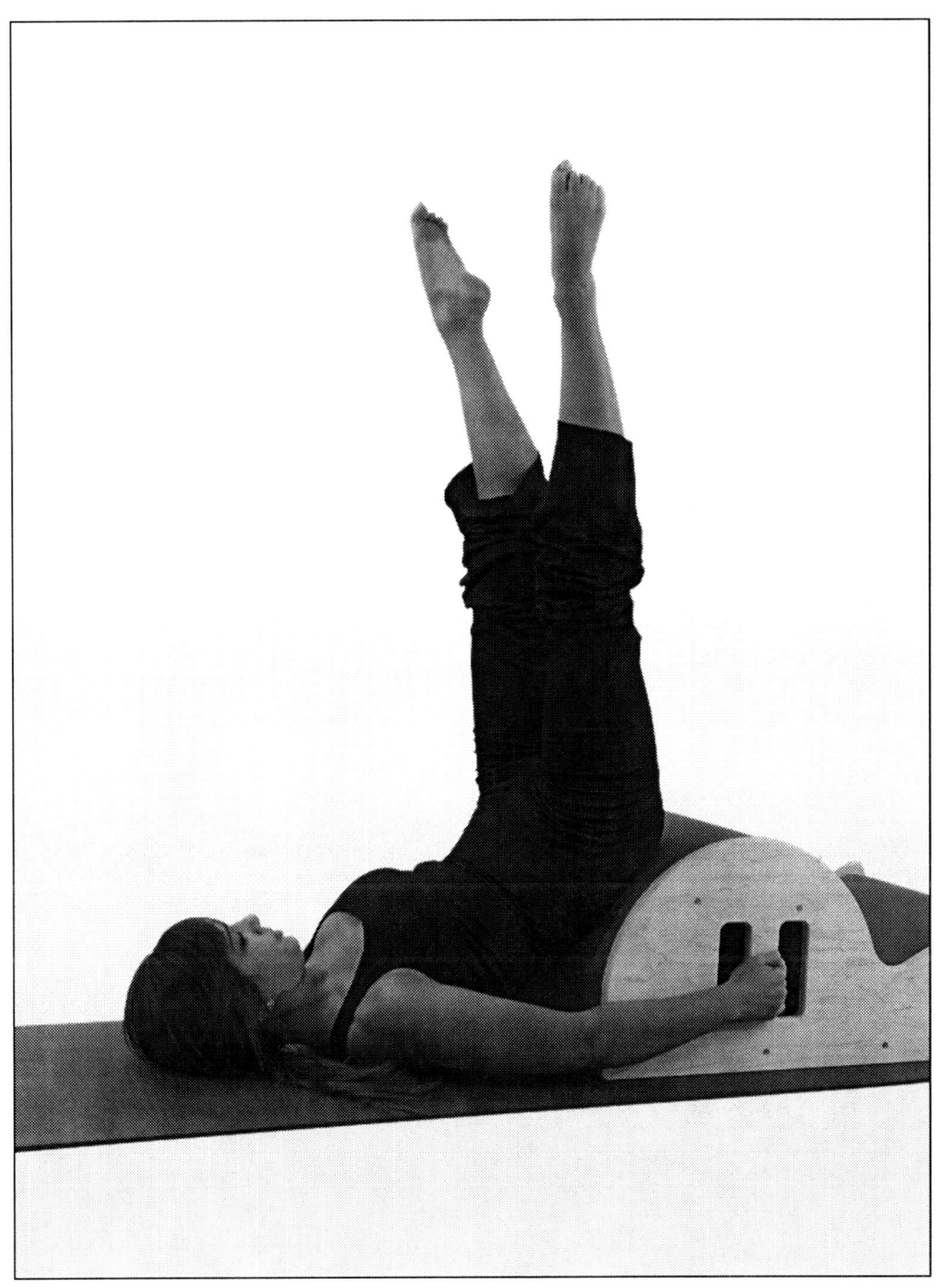

Scissors

Category: Hip mobility; disassociation of hip and spinal movement

Benefits: This exercise will improve the mobility of the hips and the stability of the pelvis.

Set-Up: Lie supine with your buttocks against the barrel. Draw your knees to your chest as you pull the barrel under you to support your low back. Hold the side handles as you lengthen your neck and extend your legs up in neutral.

Movement: While holding the handles and maintaining contact with the barrel for spine support, flex one hip as you extend the other. Attempt to keep the knees fully extended and the ribs in line with the ASIS. Hold this position for a few seconds while reaching long through the arches, and then switch the leg position. Continue for the desired repetitions, and then draw both knees to your chest to push the barrel away.

Cues:

- Reach long out of your leg.
- Relax your neck, and reach long out of the top back of your head.
- Keep the bottom of your sacrum against the barrel to maintain a posterior tilt of the pelvis.
- Keep sinking your navel to your spine.

Modification: Bend the knees slightly, and continue to move from the hip.

Breathing: Alternate your inhale and exhale as you switch the position of the legs like scissors.

Repetitions: 5 to 8

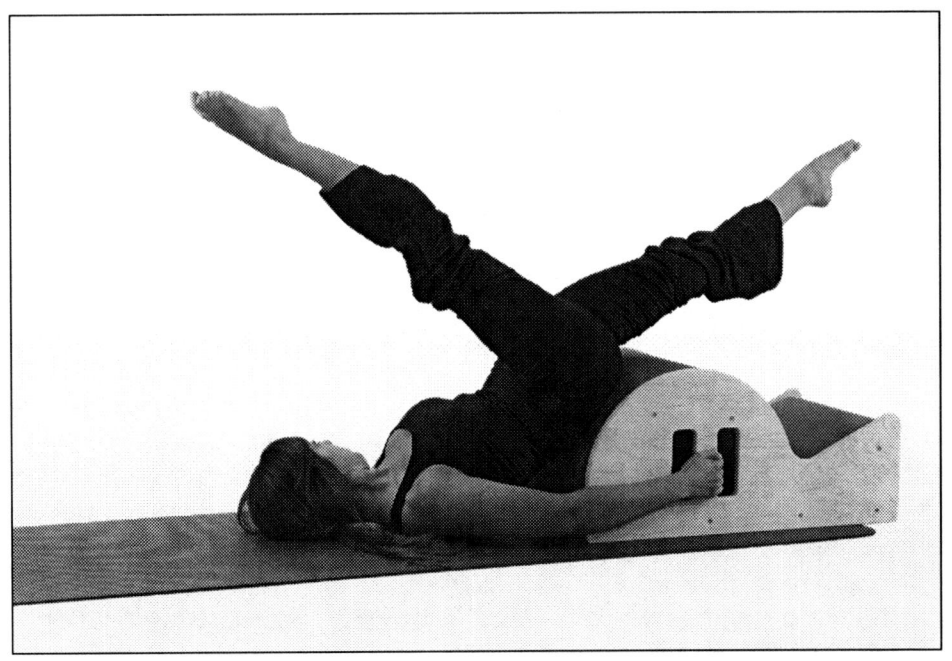
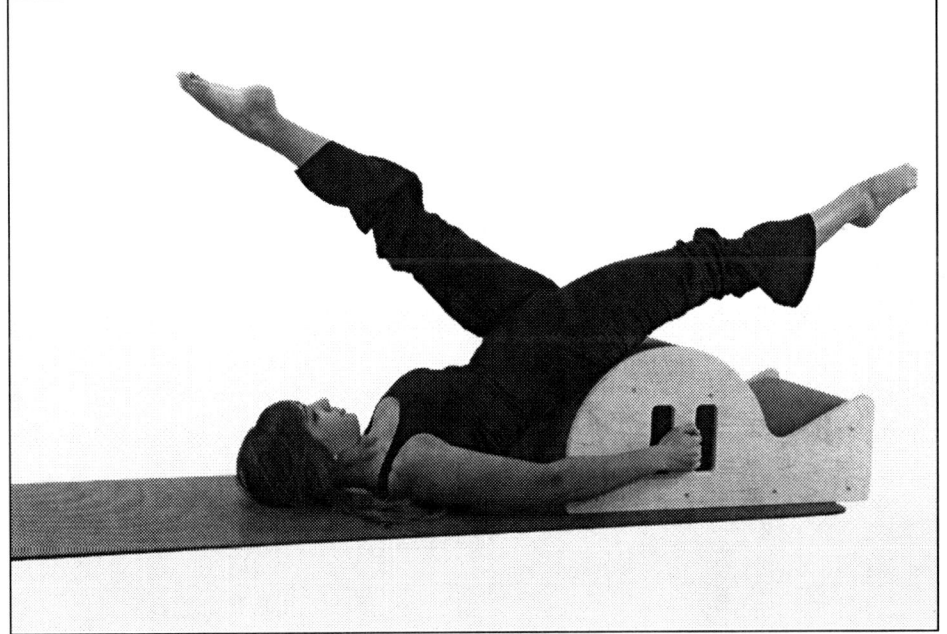

Helicopter

Category: Hip mobility; disassociation of hip and spinal movement

Benefits: This exercise will improve the mobility of the hips and the stability of the pelvis.

Set-Up: Lie supine with your buttocks against the barrel. Draw your knees to your chest as you pull the barrel under you to support your lower back. Hold the side handles as you lengthen your neck and extend your legs up in Pilates "V."

Movement: While holding the handles and maintaining contact with the barrel for spine support, flex one hip as you extend the other. Attempt to keep your knees fully extended and your ribs in line with your ASIS. Hold this position for a few seconds while reaching long through the arches, and then rotate the hips outward into a straddle. Be sure to keep the pelvis aligned and the sacrum on the barrel. Hold for a moment, and then continue around the circle into the scissor position. Hold for a moment, and then reverse to helicopter in the opposite direction. Move slowly as rapid movement of the legs could irritate the pelvic joints or pull the groin. Continue for the desired repetitions, and then draw both knees to your chest to push the barrel away.

Cues:

- Reach long out of your legs.
- Relax your neck, and reach long out of the top back of your head.
- Keep the bottom of your sacrum against the barrel to maintain lumbar support.
- Keep sinking your navel to your spine.
- Do not allow your pelvis to slip into a posterior tilt.

Modification: Bend your knees slightly, and continue to move from your hip.

Breathing: Alternate your inhale and exhale as you switch the position of the legs from scissor to straddle.

Repetitions: 5 to 8

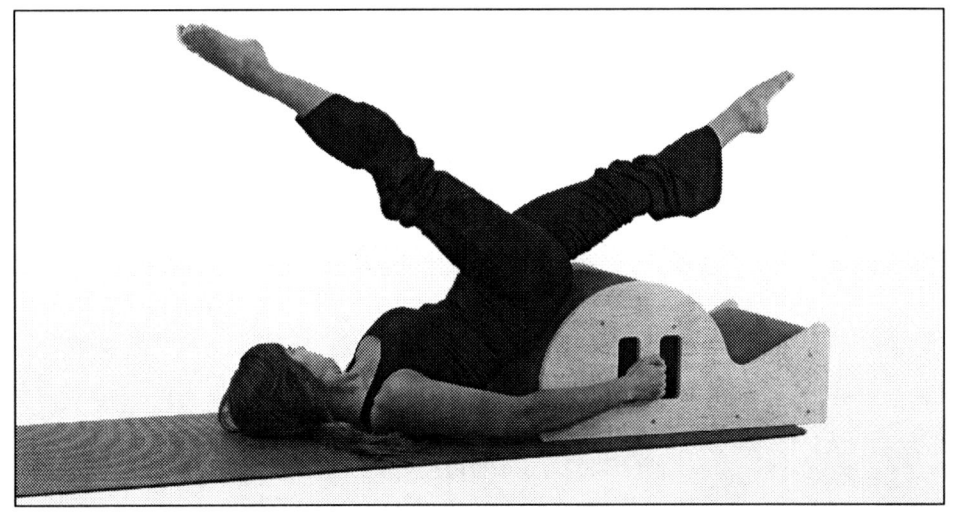
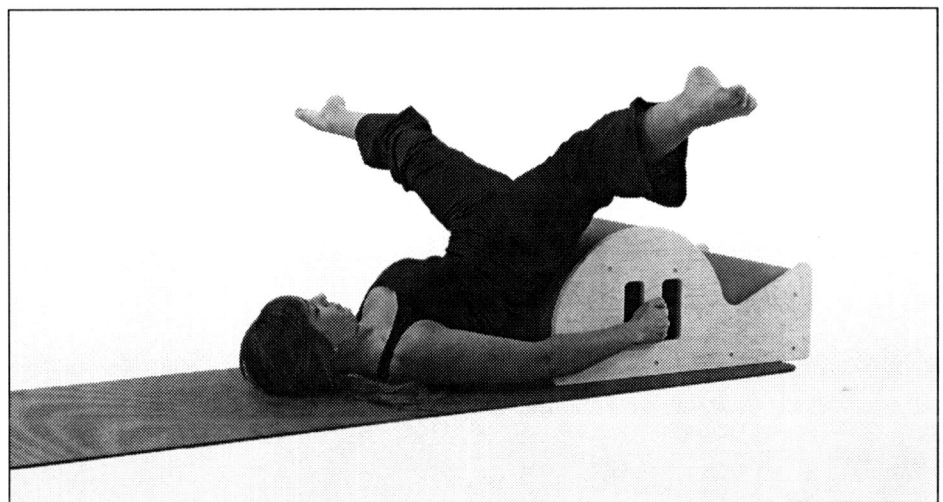
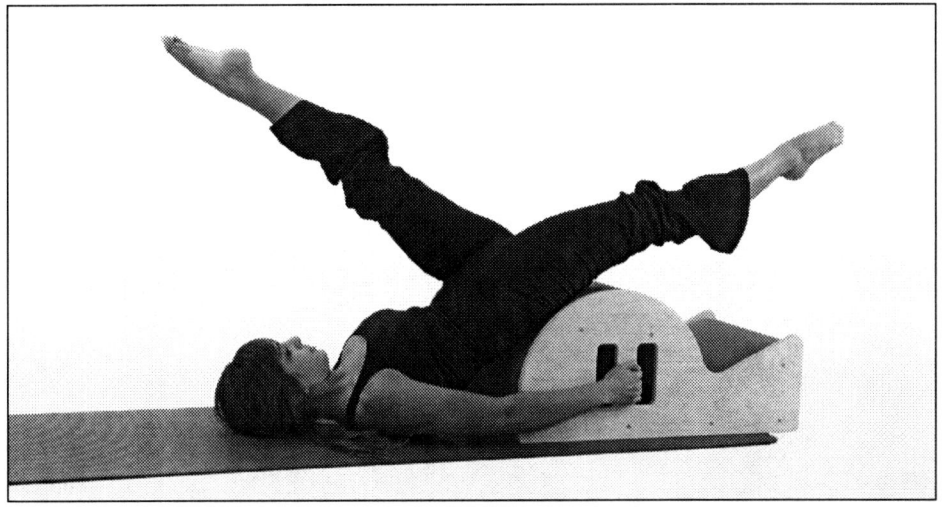

Walking

Category: Hip mobility; disassociation of hip and spinal movement

Benefits: This exercise will improve the mobility of the hips, control of the pelvis, and core stability.

Set-Up: Lie supine with your buttocks against the barrel. Draw your knees to your chest as you pull the barrel under you to support your lower back. Hold the side handles as you lengthen your neck and extend your legs with your hips in a neutral position.

Movement: While holding the handles and keeping contact with the barrel for spine support, alternate the legs in a small walking motion. Continue this motion as you walk from the ceiling down toward the mat and then back up to the ceiling. Repeat for the desired repetitions, and then draw your knees to your chest to push the barrel away.

Cues:

- Reach long out of your legs.
- Relax your neck, and reach long out of the top back of your head.
- Keep the bottom of your sacrum against the barrel to maintain lumbar support.
- Keep your hip in neutral rotation.

Modification: Walk at just one position in the range of motion.

Breathing: Inhale and exhale smoothly as you perform the walking motion. On the exhale, reinforce the navel drawing into the barrel.

Repetitions: 5 to 8

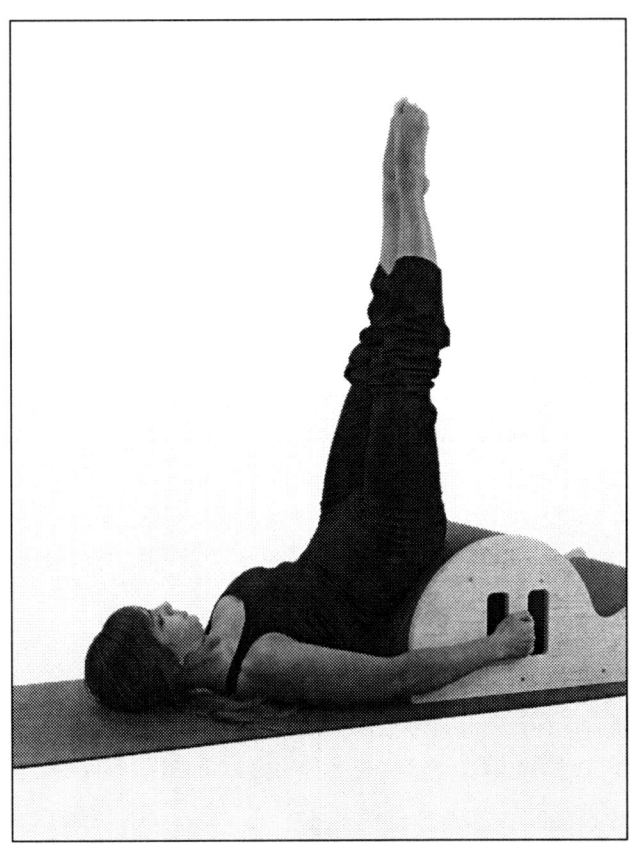

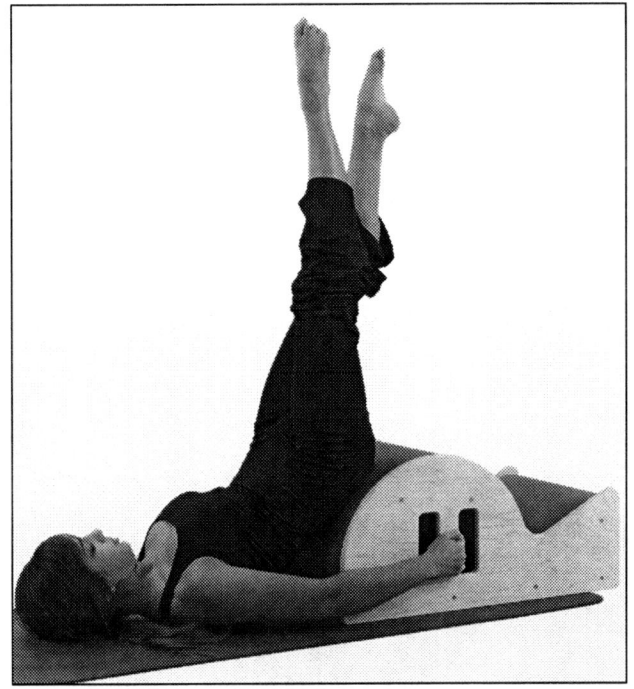

Bicycle

Category: Hip mobility; disassociation of hip and spinal movement

Benefits: This exercise will improve the mobility of the hips and the stability of the pelvis. It is especially useful for gently lengthening the hip flexors.

Set-Up: Lie supine with your buttocks against the barrel. Draw your knees to your chest as you pull the barrel under you to support your lower back. Hold the side handles as you lengthen your neck and extend one leg to the ceiling and one leg out above the floor. Position your hips in neutral rotation.

Movement: Begin by bending the knee of the lower leg and drawing the knee toward the chest while lowering the straight leg toward the edge of the spine corrector seat. Continue to hold the handles and keep contact with the barrel for spine support. Repeat these motions to finish the cycle and continue for the desired repetitions.

Cues:

- Reach long out of your legs.
- Relax your neck, and reach long out of the top back of your head.
- Keep the bottom of your sacrum against the barrel to maintain lumbar support.
- Maintain knee and second toe alignment.

Variation: Add interest by performing the exercise with flexed feet. To open the hip, hold the position when the lower leg is flexed at the knee, and reach the toes to the very edge of the spine corrector seat.

Breathing: Inhale and exhale smoothly as you perform the cycling motion. On the exhale, reinforce the navel drawing into the barrel.

Repetitions: 5 to 8

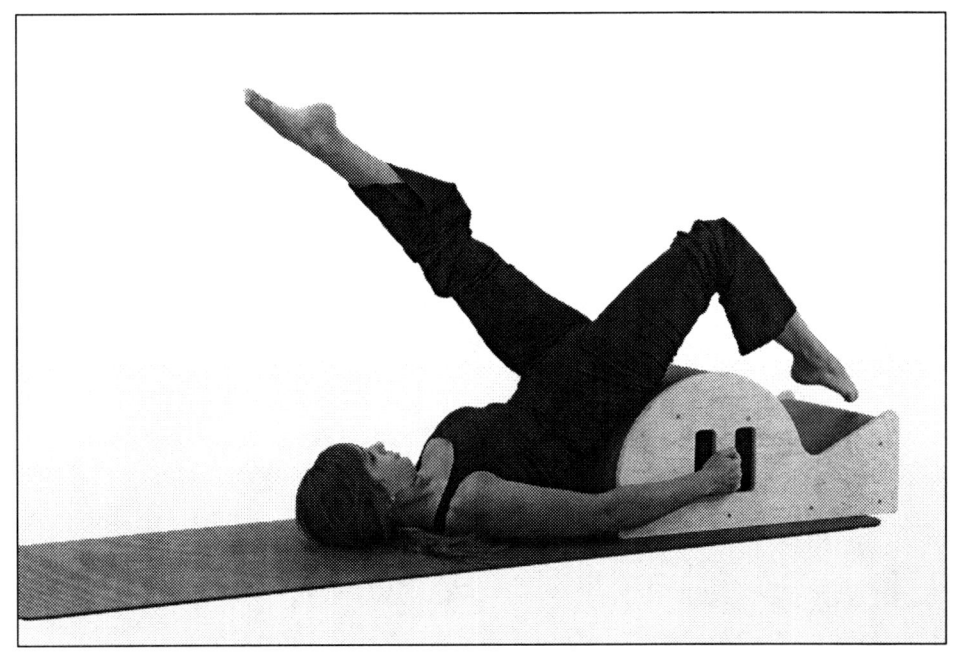

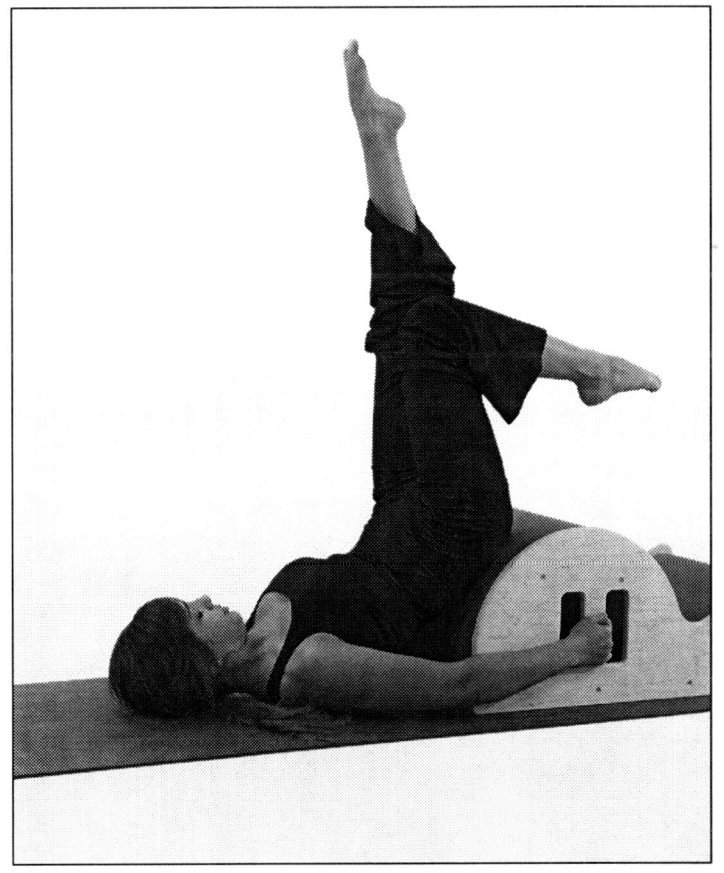

103

Beats

Category: Hip mobility; disassociation of hip and spinal movement

Benefits: This exercise will improve hip-adductor and pelvic-floor strength and endurance.

Set-Up: Lie supine with your buttocks against the barrel. Draw your knees to your chest as you pull the barrel under you to support your lower back. Hold the side handles as you lengthen your neck and extend your legs up in outward rotation.

Movement: While holding the handles and keeping contact with the barrel for spine support, abduct the legs, and begin to beat the heels toward one another. Stop the heels from hitting one another at about 1 centimeter apart. The motion should be fast and powerful.

Cues:

- Reach long out of your legs.
- Relax your neck, and reach long out of the top back of your head.
- Keep the bottom of your sacrum against the barrel to maintain lumbar support.
- Draw up and in with your inner thighs, and zip and wrap at your hips.

Variation: Perform this exercise with either a flexed or pointed foot. Avoid sickling at the foot.

Breathing: Inhale and exhale smoothly as you perform the beats. Reinforce the navel to spine each time that you exhale.

Repetitions: 5 to 8

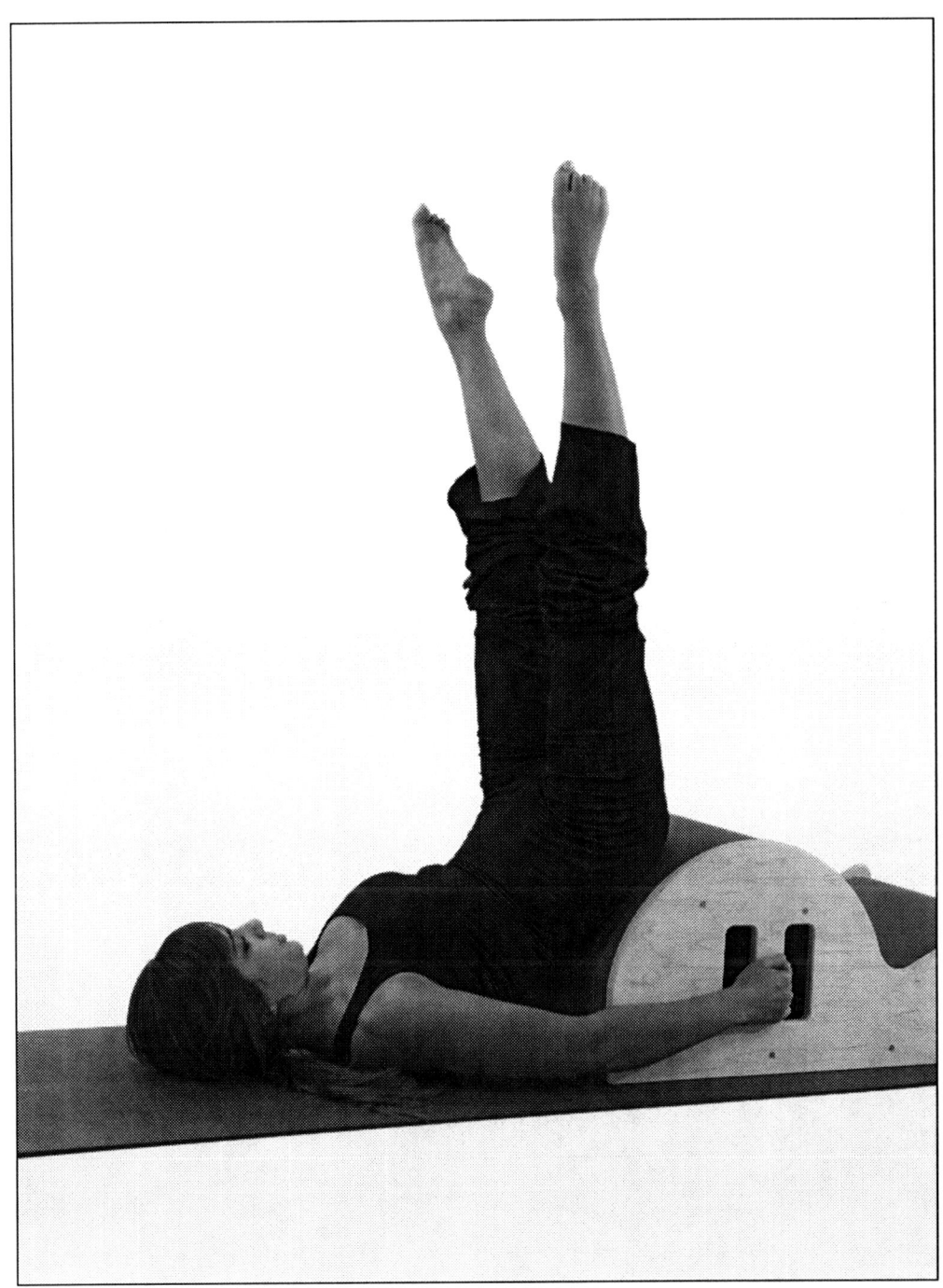

Rolling In and Out

Category: Lumbar mobility; disassociation of hip and spinal movement

Benefits: This exercise will improve the mobility of the lumbar spine and core stability.

Set-Up: Lie supine with your buttocks against the barrel. Draw your knees to your chest as you pull the barrel under you to support your lower back. Hold the side handles as you lengthen your neck.

Movement: While holding the handles and maintaining contact with the barrel for spine support, draw your knees toward your right ear. Then rock your knees toward your left ear. Repeat this motion for the desired repetitions, and then come to center before you push the barrel away.

Cues:

- Keep your knees together.
- Relax your neck, and reach long out of the top back of your head.
- Keep the bottom of your sacrum against the barrel to maintain lumbar support.
- Your ribcage should be stable with no rotation.

Variations: Use a small ball between the knees to assist with the adduction of the legs and engage the pelvic-floor muscles.

Breathing: Inhale as you bring your legs down and together. Exhale as you bring your legs to your right ear. Inhale in the center, and exhale as you go toward your left ear.

Repetitions: 5 to 8

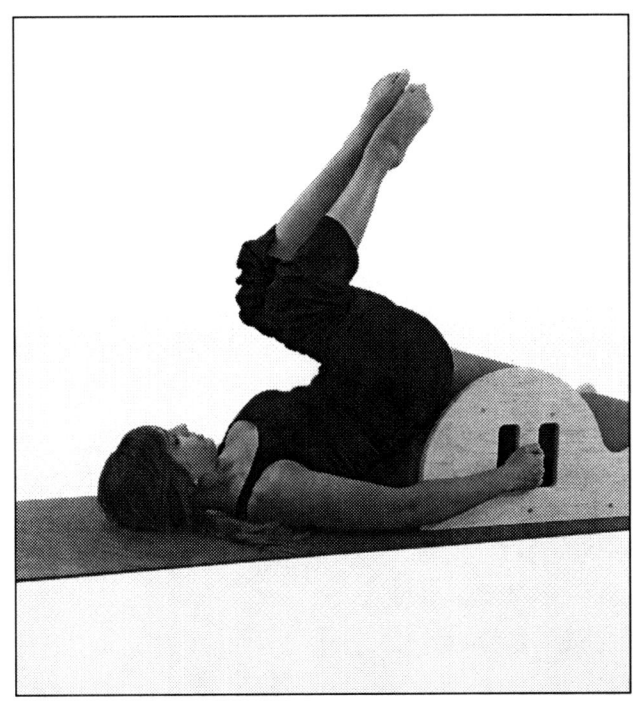

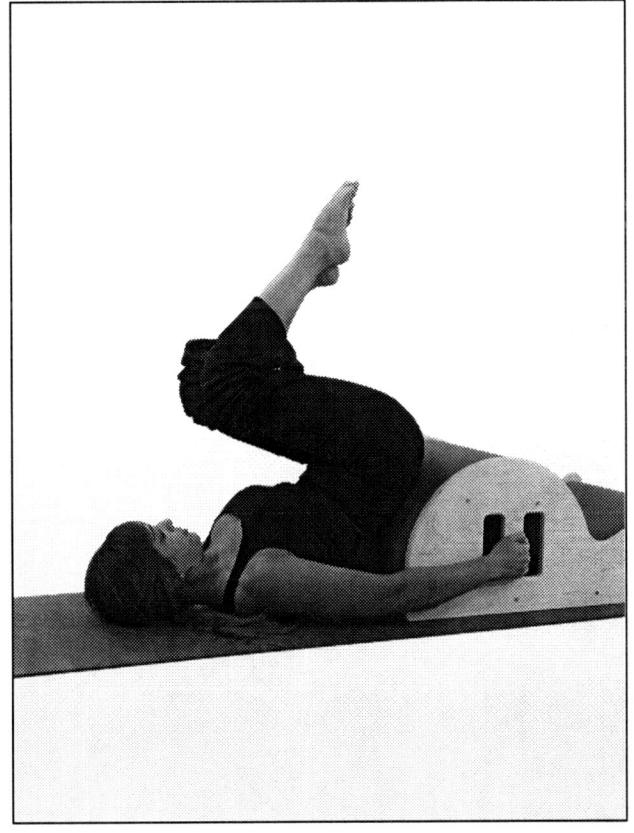

Stretch With Bar

Category: Glenohumeral mobility; scapular stability

Benefits: This exercise will improve the stability of the shoulder girdle, open the chest, and balance the cervical muscles.

Set-Up: Sit with your coccyx on the edge of the barrel. Your legs should be straight, and your body will lie back over the barrel. Keep your gaze toward your feet, and lengthen the back of your neck. Align your ASIS and your 10th rib angle. Zip and wrap your legs. Your arms should be extended along your sides holding the dowel rod or Pilates ring.

Movement: Reach your arms up and overhead while maintaining the pelvis and ribs against the barrel. Return your arms to your sides. Repeat for the desired repetitions.

Cues:

- Reach long out of your shoulders.
- Draw your ribs into the barrel.
- Keep the bottom of your coccyx against the barrel to maintain lumbar extension and support.

Progression: You may use small hand weights for this exercise or a weighted bar.

Repetitions: 5 to 8

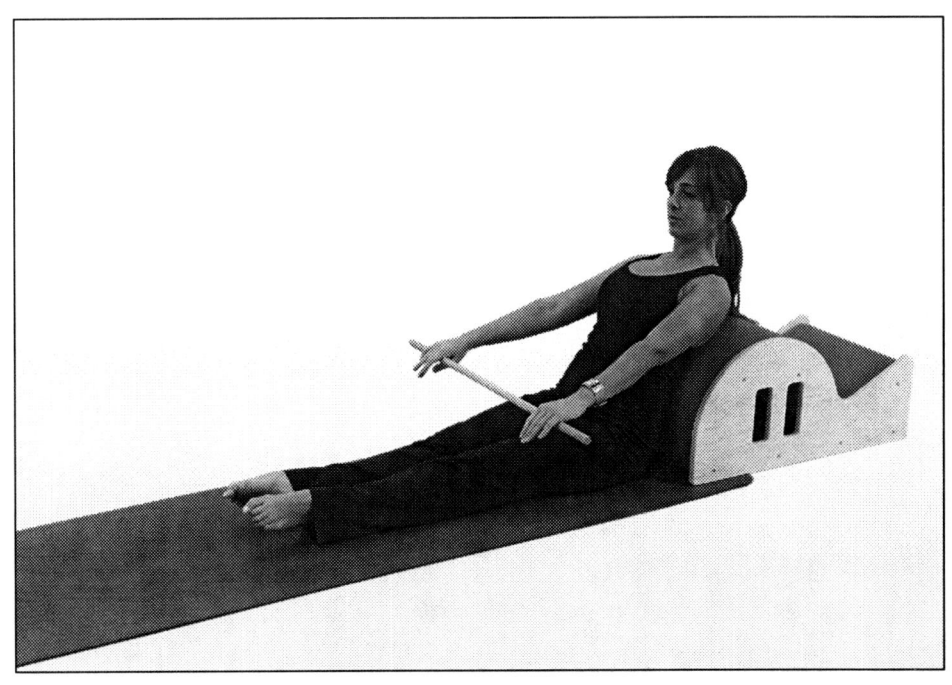

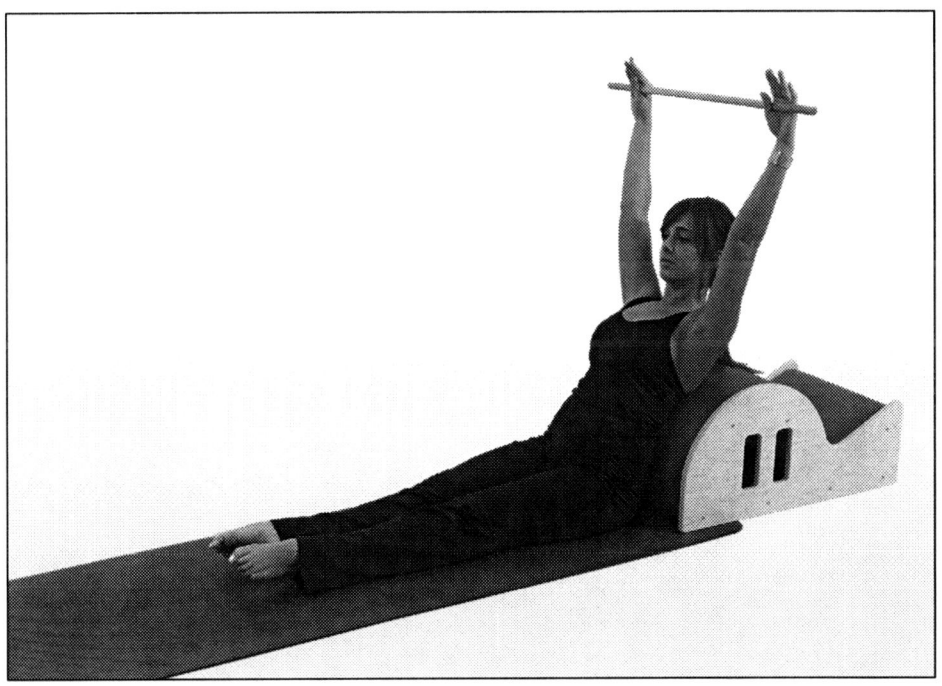

Teaser

Category: Core strengthening

Benefits: This exercise will improve the stability of the core, lengthen the hamstrings, and strengthen the hip flexors.

Set-Up: Sit in the hollow section of the barrel facing the barrel end. Your arms and legs should be up in the teaser position.

Movement: Roll back over the edge of the seat while keeping the legs up in Pilates "V" and raising your arms overhead. Return to the teaser position. Repeat for the desired repetitions.

Cues:

- Reach long out of your legs.
- Draw your navel to your spine as you exhale.
- Be sure that your body only goes back as far as you can control.

Modification: Try keeping the upper body in the teaser position while lowering the legs or bend the knees to shorten the lever.

Breathing: Inhale as you roll back, and exhale as you return to the teaser position.

Repetitions: 5 to 8

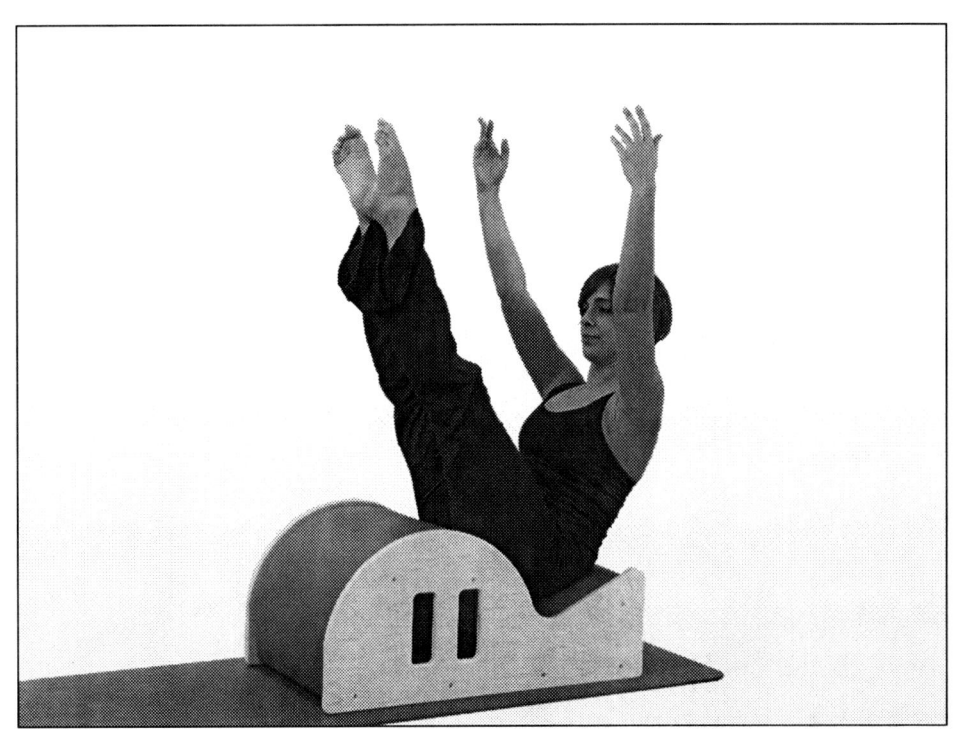
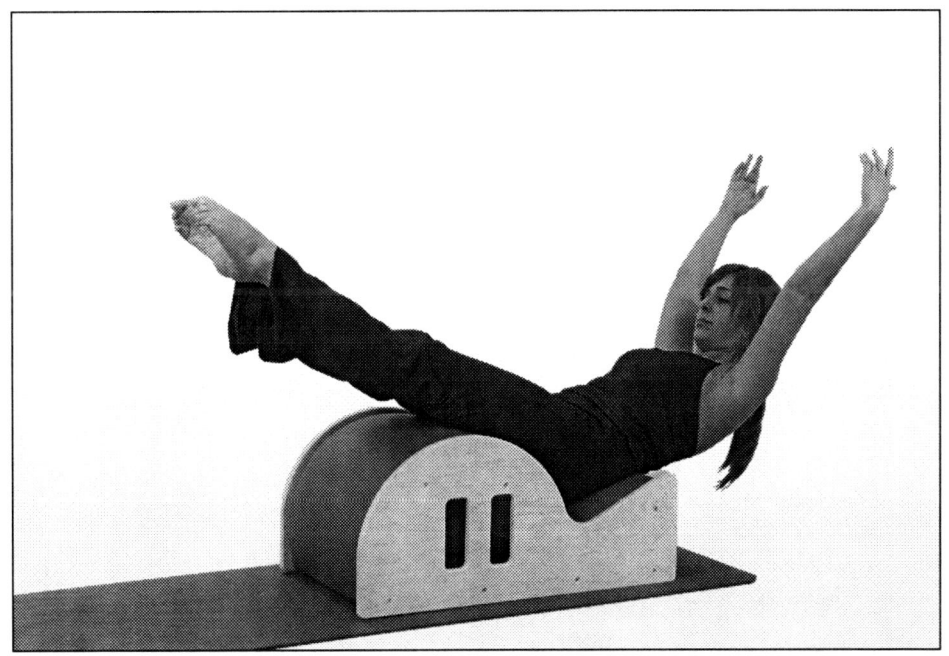

Swan

Category: Spinal extension; hip extension

Benefits: This exercise will improve the stability of the core, strengthen the paraspinal muscles and the hip extensors, and disassociate hip and spinal movement.

Set-Up: Lie prone facing the barrel end with your abdomen over the hump of the barrel. This will be a personal position where you are able to find your point of balance. Extend your legs out long in Pilates "V."

Movement: Reach long through the top of your head and extend your spine. Return to the start position, and repeat for the desired repetitions.

Cues:

- Reach long out of your legs.
- Draw your navel to your spine as you exhale.
- Keep your ear in line with your ribs as you swan.

Variation: Try this exercise holding the ring between the ankles.

Breathing: Inhale as you reach long through the top of your head and extend your spine. Exhale as you return to the start position.

Repetitions: 5 to 8

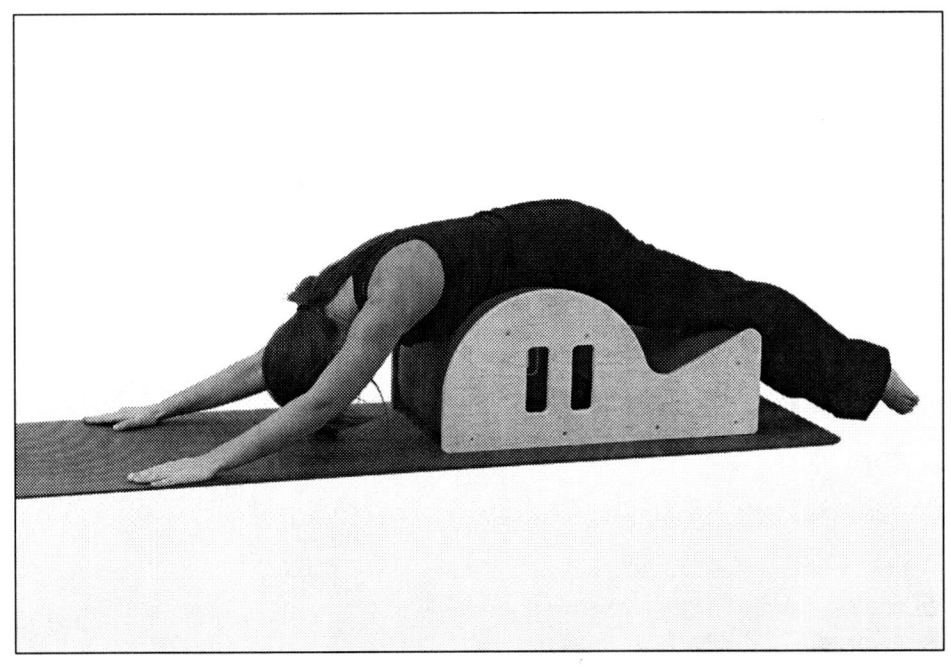
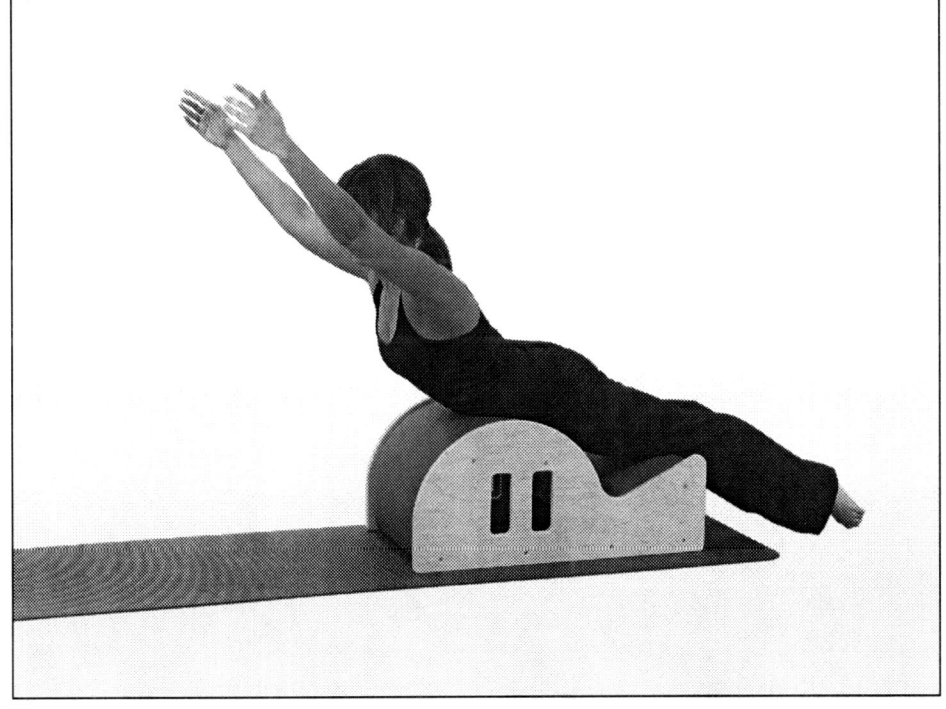

Hip Circles

Category: Core strengthening

Benefits: This exercise will improve the stability of the core, lengthen the hamstrings, and strengthen the hip flexors.

Set-Up: Sit in the hollow section of the barrel facing the barrel end. Your legs should be up in teaser position in Pilates "V." Your hands are holding the edge of the seat to assist in keeping your chest open.

Movement: Circle the legs from your right ear to your left ear for the desired repetitions, and then reverse.

Cues:

- Reach long out of your legs.
- Draw your navel to your spine as you exhale.
- Be sure that your legs only move in a range that you can control.
- Keep the back tall and the shoulders wide.

Variation: Try this exercise holding the ring between the ankles.

Breathing: Inhale as you start one side of the circle, and exhale as you complete the circle.

Repetitions: 5 to 8

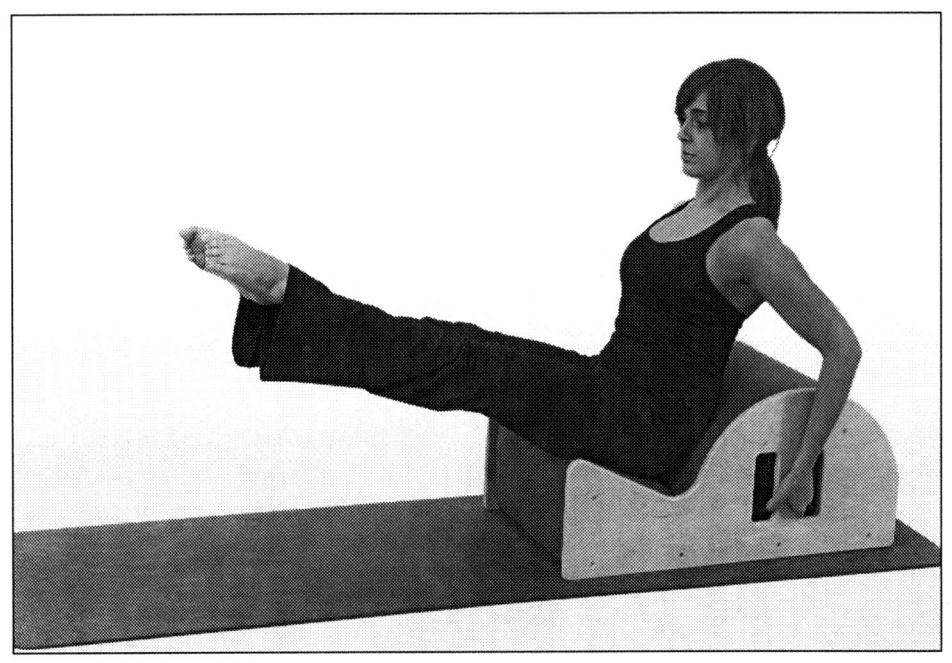
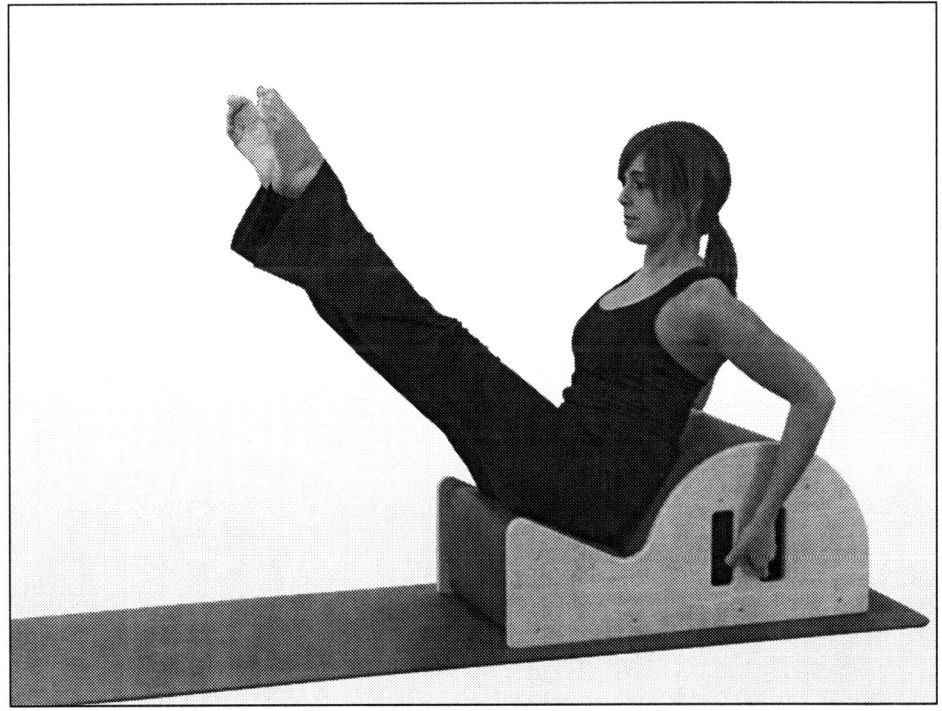

115

Mermaid

Category: Spinal flexibility; core strengthening; hip mobility

Benefits: This exercise will improve stability of the core, strengthen the paraspinal muscles and the obliques, strengthen the hip abductors, and improve hip rotation.

Set-Up: Sit in the hollow of the barrel, facing the side with one hip in internal rotation and one hip in external rotation. Allow the front leg to come down in front of the side of the barrel while aligning your ASIS with the wall in front of you. Sit tall with your arms extended out from your shoulders.

Movement: Begin by reaching away from the hump of the barrel, and then reach over the hump to form a "C" curve. Pause to stretch, and then draw the navel to the spine as you sit up. Take a moment to stack the spine, and then reach the ribcage over the barrel to side bend. Repeat for the desired repetitions.

Cues:

- Reach your ischial tuberosities toward the seat of the spine corrector.
- Keep your body in line with the wall in front of you.
- Draw your navel to your spine as you exhale.
- Pull yourself up with your top hand. Do not push with the bottom hand.

Modification: Try this exercise while supported by your elbow on the hump of the barrel.

Breathing: Inhale to prepare, and exhale as you lift yourself up, drawing the navel to the spine. Inhale at the top of the motion, and exhale as you return to the hump of the barrel with control.

Repetitions: 5 to 8

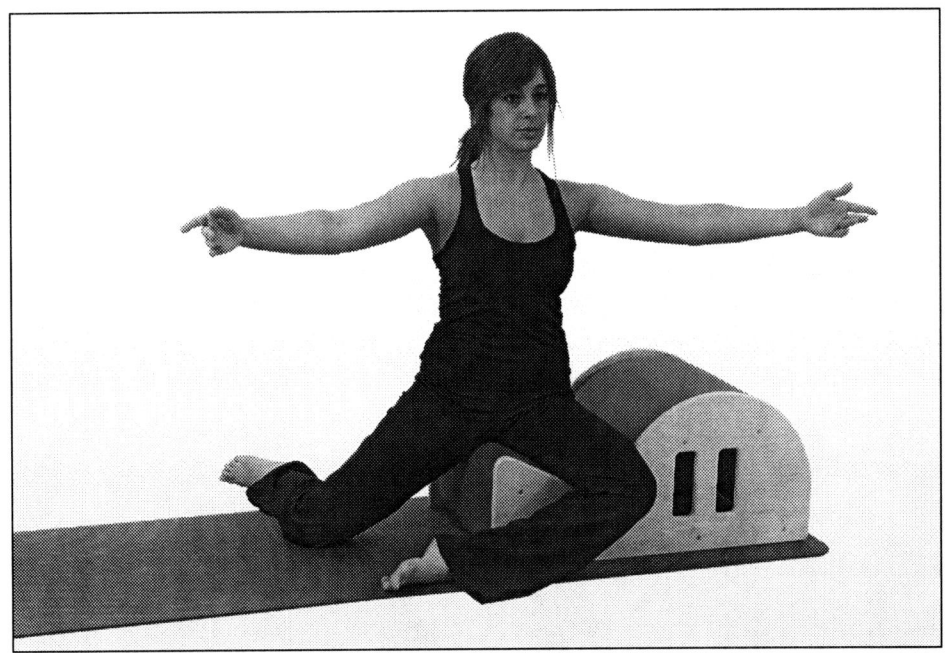
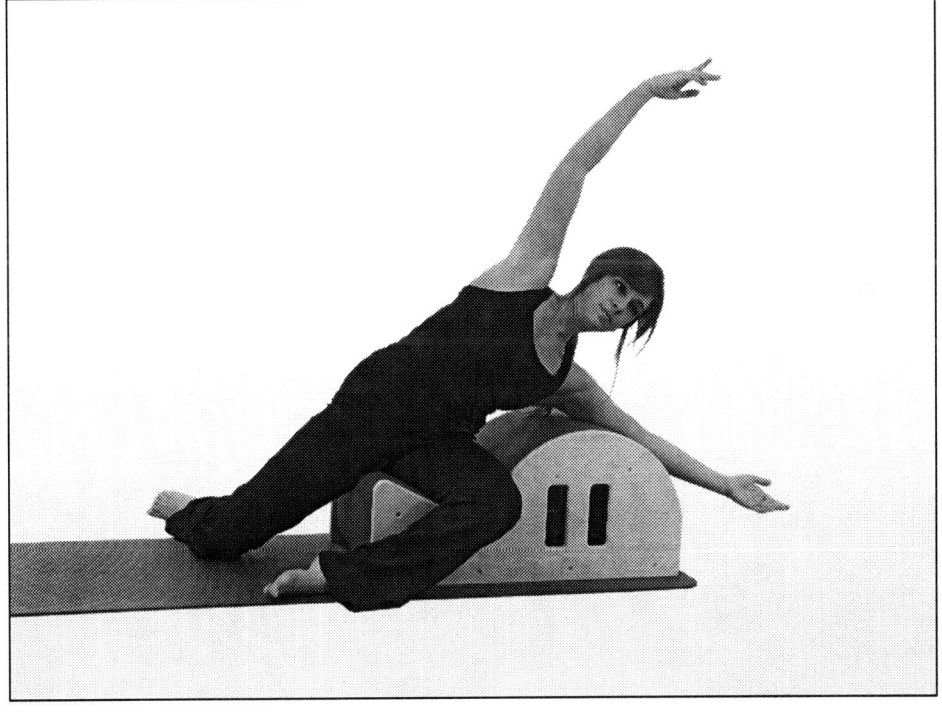

Mermaid Legs

Category: Hip and core strengthening; hip mobility

Benefits: This exercise will improve the stability of the core, strengthen the quadratus lumborum and the obliques, strengthen the hip abductors, and improve hip rotation.

Set-Up: Sit in the hollow of the barrel, facing the side with one hip in internal rotation and one hip in external rotation. Allow your front leg to come down in front of the side of the barrel while aligning your ASIS with the wall in front of you. Position your elbow on the hump of the barrel, and draw the shoulder blade down the back while engaging the external oblique.

Movement: While maintaining the set-up position, abduct your leg without any hip rotation. Repeat for the desired repetitions, and then change sides.

Cues:

- Reach your ischial tuberosities toward the seat of the spine corrector.
- Keep your body in line with the wall in front of you.
- Draw your navel to your spine as you exhale.
- Maintain the ribcage position as you lift your leg.

Progression: To add challenge, extend the knee while your leg is up in abduction.

Breathing: Inhale to prepare, and exhale as you raise your leg.

Repetitions: 5 to 8

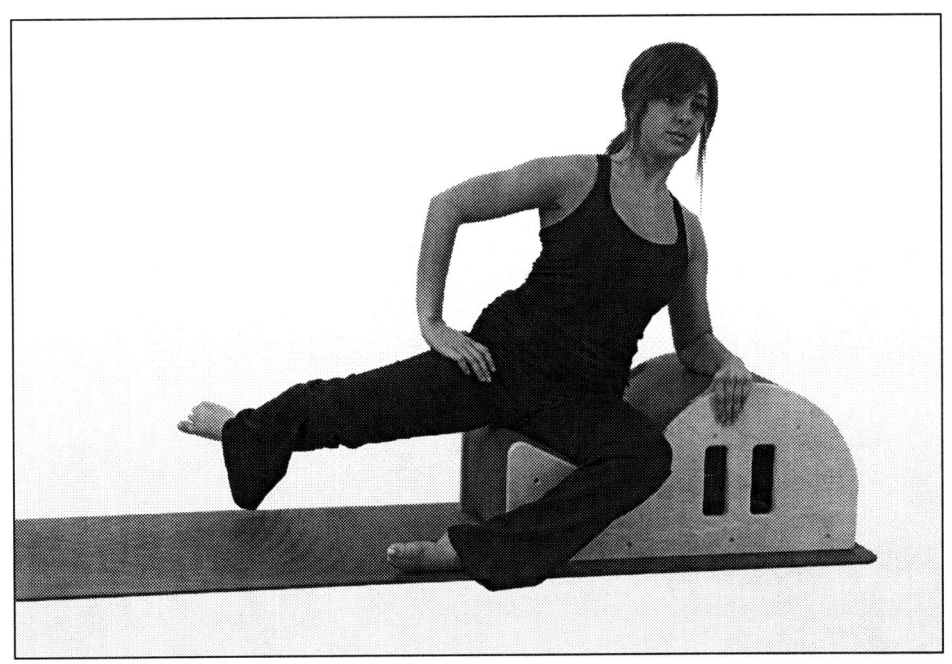

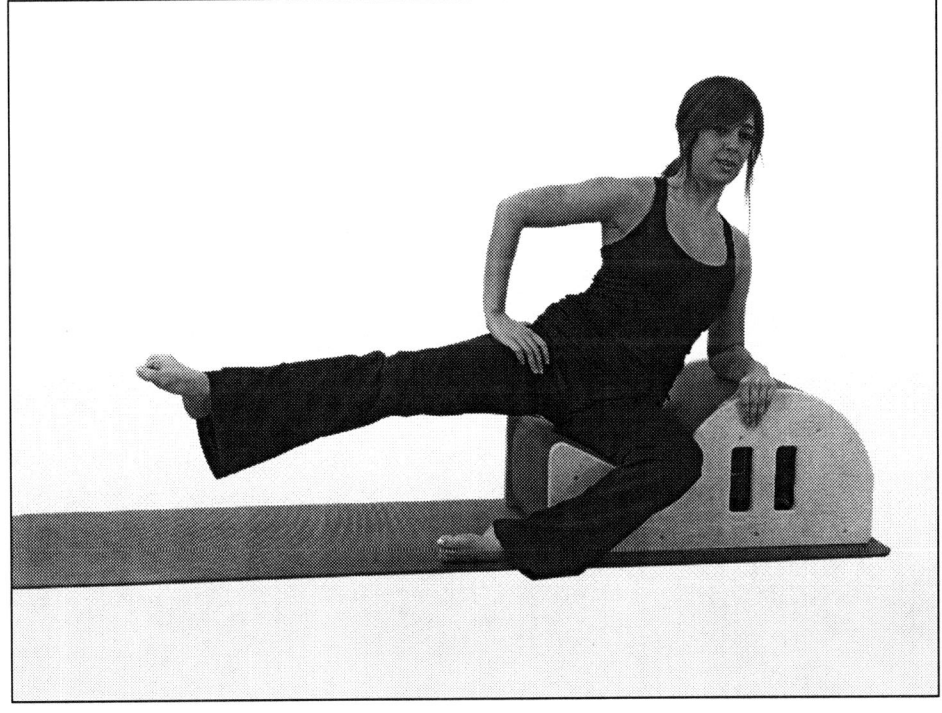

Shoulder Bridge

Category: Hip mobility; hip and back extensor strengthening

Benefits: This exercise will improve the stability of the core, strengthen the paraspinal muscles and the obliques, strengthen the hip extensors, and improve hip extension.

Set-Up: Lie supine with your buttocks against the barrel. Draw your knees to your chest as you pull the barrel under you to support your lower back. Hold the side handles as you lengthen your neck. Place your feet on the seat of the spine corrector in line with your ischial tuberosities.

Movement: Engage your gluteals, and extend your hips and spine into a bridge.

Cues:

- Keep the ribs in line with the ASIS and the knees in line with the second toe.
- Draw your navel to your spine as you exhale.

Progression: For more challenge, try this exercise with a single-leg position. Reach the non-weight-bearing leg toward the ceiling.

Modification: If you are shorter, you may need to use the baby arc for this exercise.

Breathing: Inhale to prepare, and exhale as you lift yourself up, drawing the navel to the spine.

Repetitions: 5 to 8

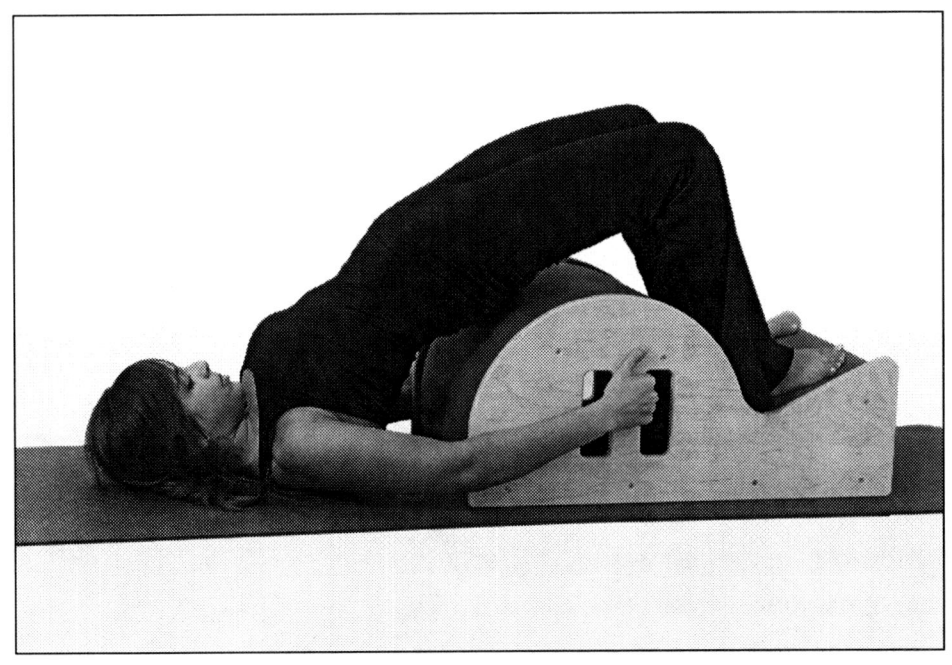

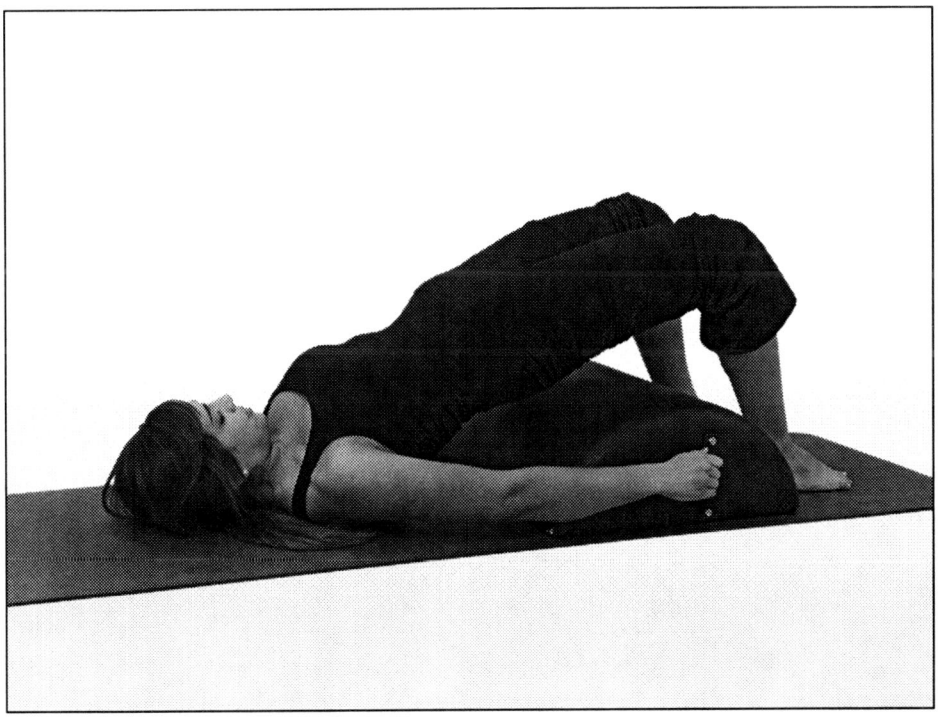

Swimming

Category: Spinal extension; hip extension

Benefits: This exercise will improve the stability of the core, strengthen the paraspinal muscles and the hip extensors, and will disassociate hip and spinal movement.

Set-Up: Lie prone, facing the barrel end with your abdomen over the hump of the barrel. This will be a personal position where you are able to find your point of balance. Extend your legs out long in Pilates "V."

Movement: Reach long through the top of your head, while you reach one arm and the opposite leg. Repeat with your other side, and alternate for the desired repetitions.

Cues:

- Reach long out of your legs and shoulders.
- Draw your navel to your spine as you exhale.
- Keep your ear in line with your ribs.
- Do not allow your pelvis to rock from side to side or your lumbar spine to extend.

Breathing: Inhale as you reach arm and leg, and exhale as you return to the start position.

Variations: Try changing the speed with which you switch sides. You may add small weights to the arms.

Repetitions: 5 to 8

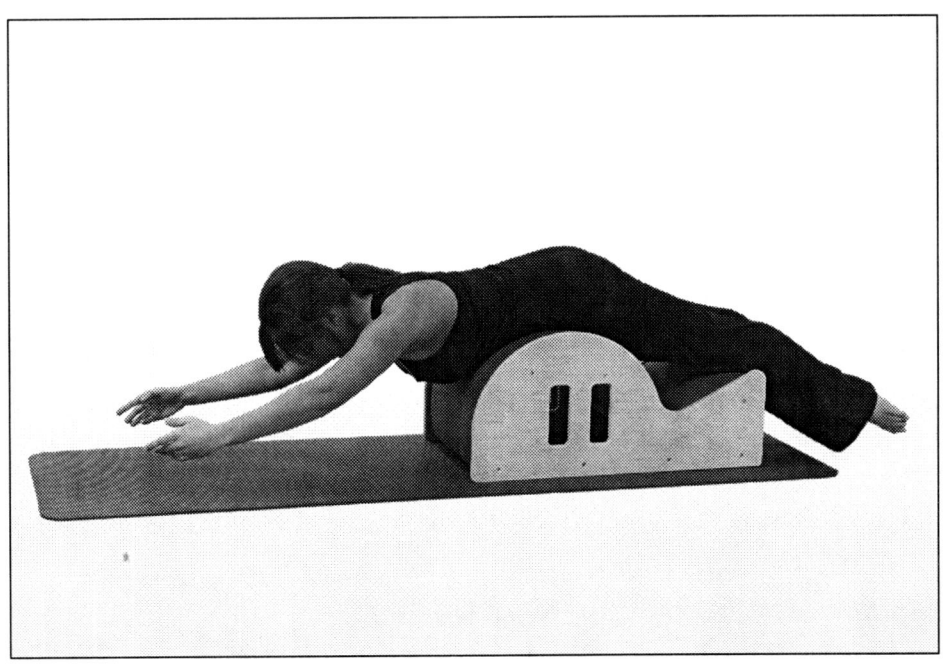

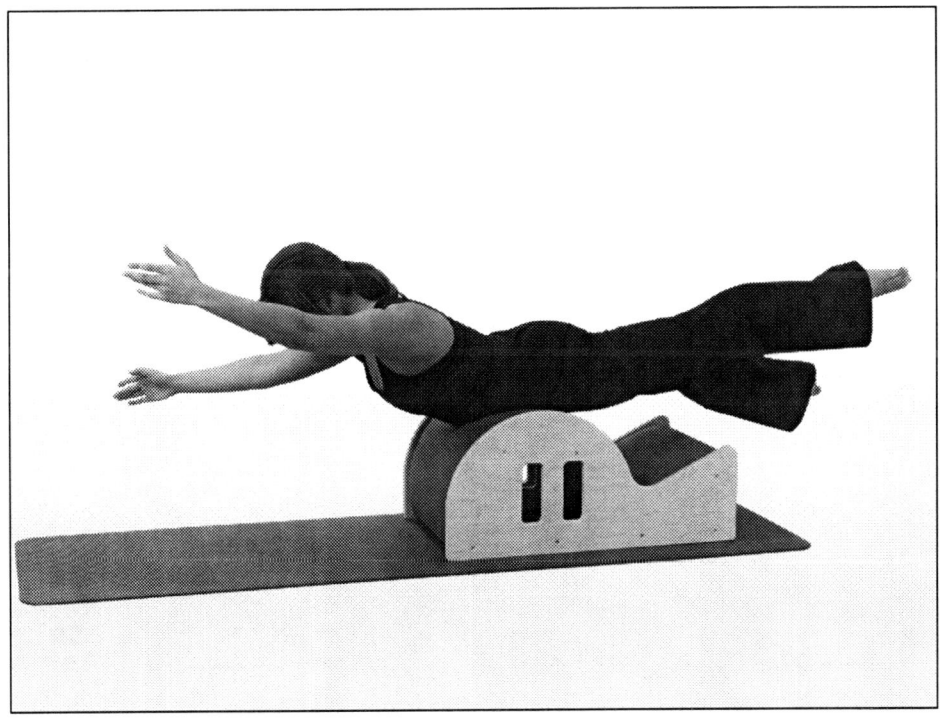

Seated Twist

Category: Core strengthening; hip and spine disassociation

Benefits: This exercise will improve the stability of the core and pelvis, and increase the flexibility of the spine.

Set-Up: Sit in the hollow section of the barrel facing the barrel end. Place your legs in abduction and external rotation with your feet flat on the floor knees bent. Reach your arms out to the sides in a position of scaption.

Movement: Rotate your spine to one side without moving your pelvis or legs. Return to the center, and grow tall. Continue to alternate sides for the desired repetitions.

Cues:

- Do not allow the legs or pelvis to move while you twist.
- Draw your navel to your spine as you exhale.

Variation: Add three reaches in the twist like you would on the mat.

Breathing: Inhale in the center, and exhale as you twist to each side.

Repetitions: 5 to 8

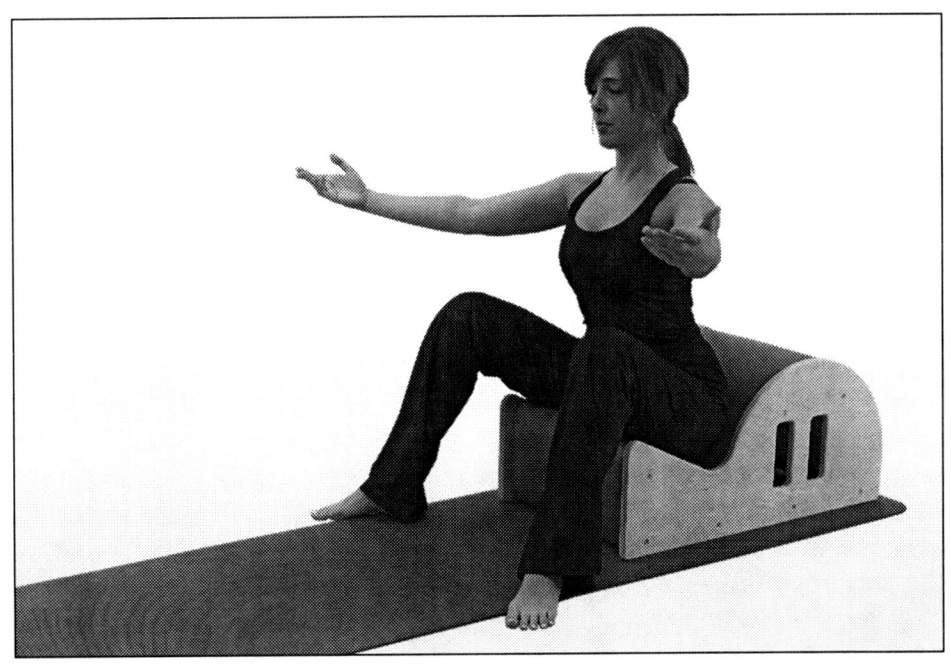
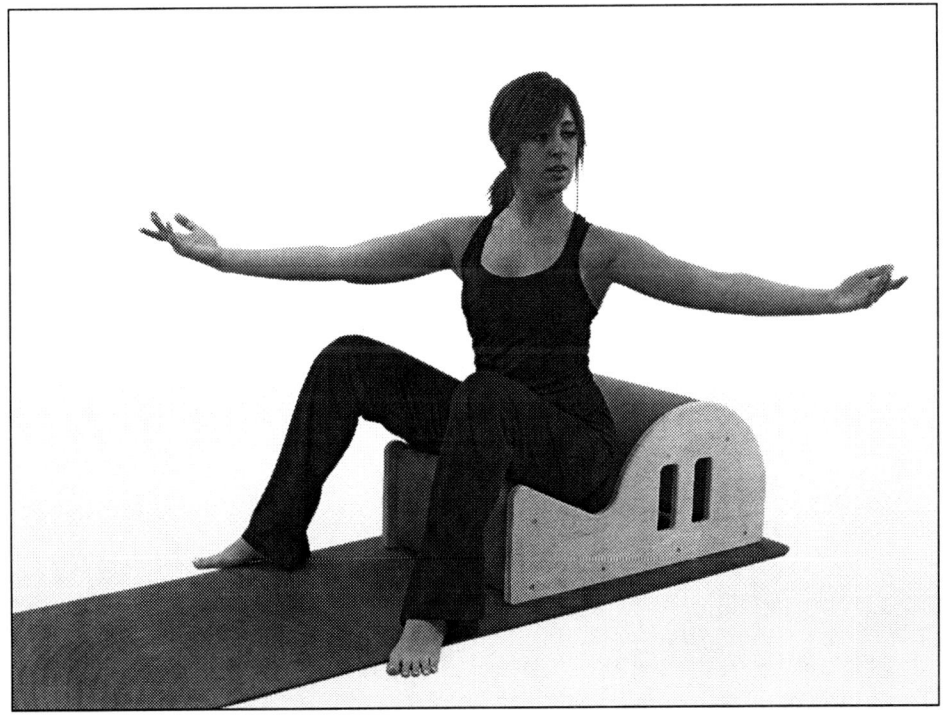

Roll-Up

Category: Spinal flexibility; core strengthening

Benefits: This exercise will improve the stability of the core, strengthen the obliques and rectus abdominis, and improve the movement of the shoulder girdle.

Set-Up: Sit in the hollow of the barrel, facing away from the barrel. Sit up tall with your shoulders over your hips and your legs in a bowl-sit position. Your arms should be extended at shoulder height.

Movement: Begin by going into a posterior tilt without collapsing your upper body. Draw your lower back into the barrel, and continue rolling back over the barrel one vertebra at a time. Be cautious with your neck as cervical extension can cause dizziness. Maintain the cervical spine at neutral, and do not extend. Once you are back over the barrel, raise the arms to frame your face while maintaining the ribcage position. Nod your chin and roll up, bringing your face through the window of your arms. Arms stay up until you have completely rolled up to the starting position. Repeat for the desired repetitions.

Cues:

- Draw your navel to your spine as you exhale.
- Imagine your body as a string of pearls being dropped one at a time and then being picked up one at a time.

Variations: Try this exercise holding the ring.

Breathing: Inhale to prepare, and exhale as you roll back. Inhale as you lift your arms overhead, and exhale as you roll up.

Repetitions: 5 to 8

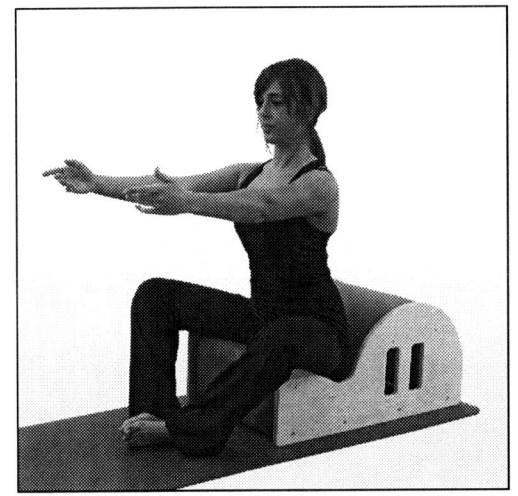
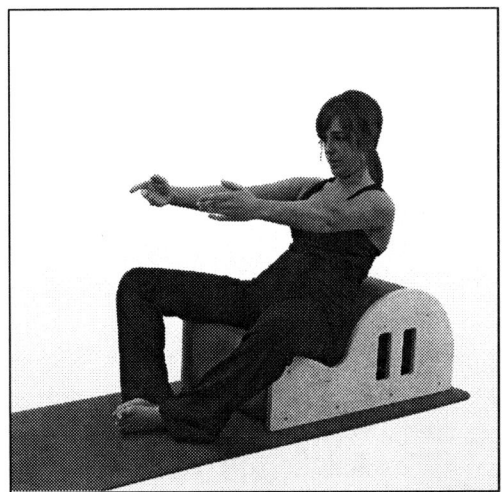
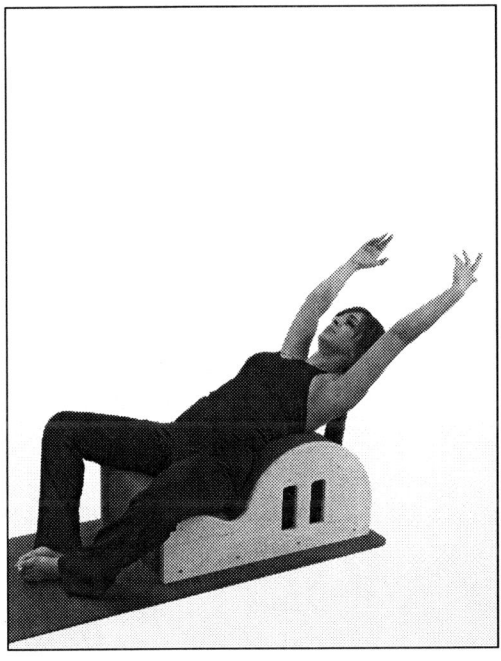
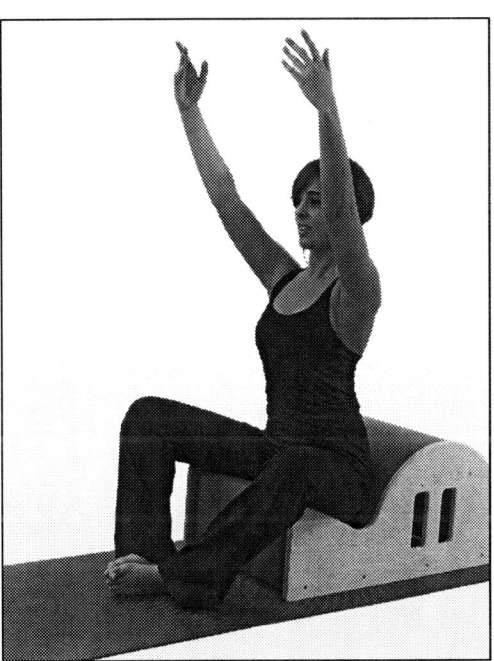

5

Small Barrel (Baby Arc)

Arm Circles

Category: Spinal mobility, especially thoracic and lumbar extension

Benefits: This exercise will improve stability of the shoulder girdle and the mobility of the thoracic and lumbar spine.

Set-Up: Lie with your upper back against the barrel. Perform a cervical nod, and reach out of the top back of your head. Extend your legs out long in outward rotation, and bring the back of the sacrum against the curve of the barrel. Your arms should be extended along your sides with your chest open.

Movement: Reach your arms up and overhead while maintaining the position against the barrel. Continue the circle around to return to your sides. Repeat for the desired repetitions, and then reverse the direction.

Cues:

- Reach long out of your shoulders.
- Draw your ribs into the barrel.
- Keep the bottom of your sacrum against the barrel to maintain lumbar extension and support.

Modification: Make the circles very small with control.

Progression: You may use small weights for this exercise or a weighted bar for just shoulder flexion and extension.

Breathing: Inhale as you reach overhead, and exhale for the remainder of the circle. To perform the opposite direction, inhale as you abduct the arms to the sides, and exhale as you return them to the start position.

Repetitions: 5 to 8

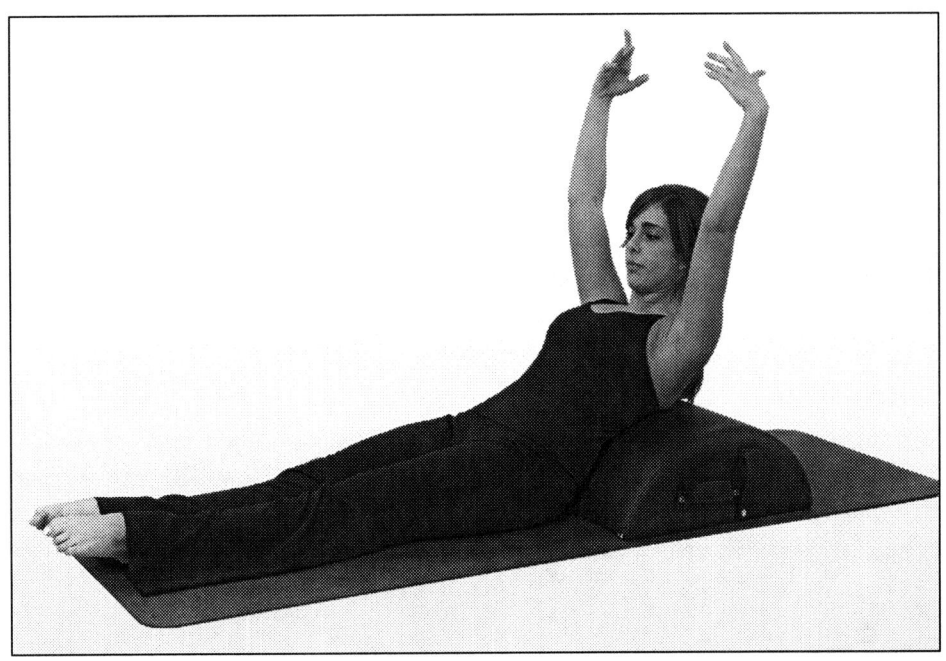
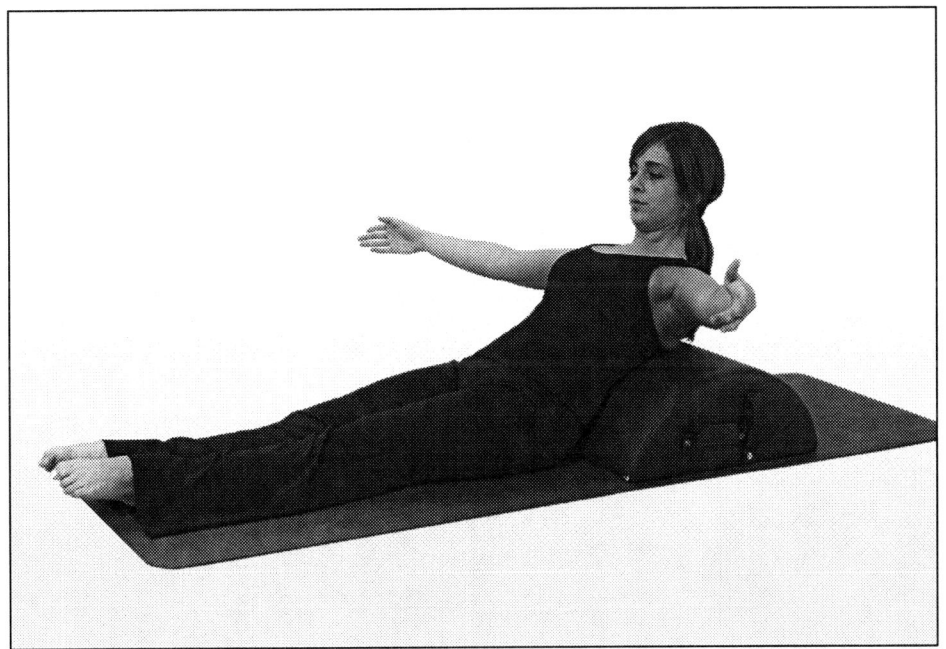

Leg Circles

Category: Hip mobility; disassociation of hip and spinal movement

Benefits: This exercise will improve the mobility of the hips and the control of the pelvis.

Set-Up: Lie supine with your buttocks against the barrel. Draw the knees to your chest as you pull the barrel under you to support your lower back. Hold the side handles as you lengthen your neck and extend your legs up in outward rotation.

Movement: While holding the handles and keeping contact with the barrel for spine support, abduct your legs and begin to circle out. Draw your legs down and together, and then bring them back to the starting position. Repeat the circles for the desired repetitions and then reverse the direction. The exercise may be done in hip outward rotation or hip neutral. Avoid hip internal rotation.

Cues:

- Reach long out of your legs.
- Relax your neck and reach long out of the top back of your head.
- Keep the bottom of your sacrum against the barrel to maintain lumbar support.

Modification: Make the circles very small with control.

Breathing: Inhale as you open the legs and draw them down and together. Exhale as you bring the legs up into the starting position. For the opposite motion, inhale as you draw the legs down, and exhale as you abduct and return to the starting position.

Repetitions: 5 to 8

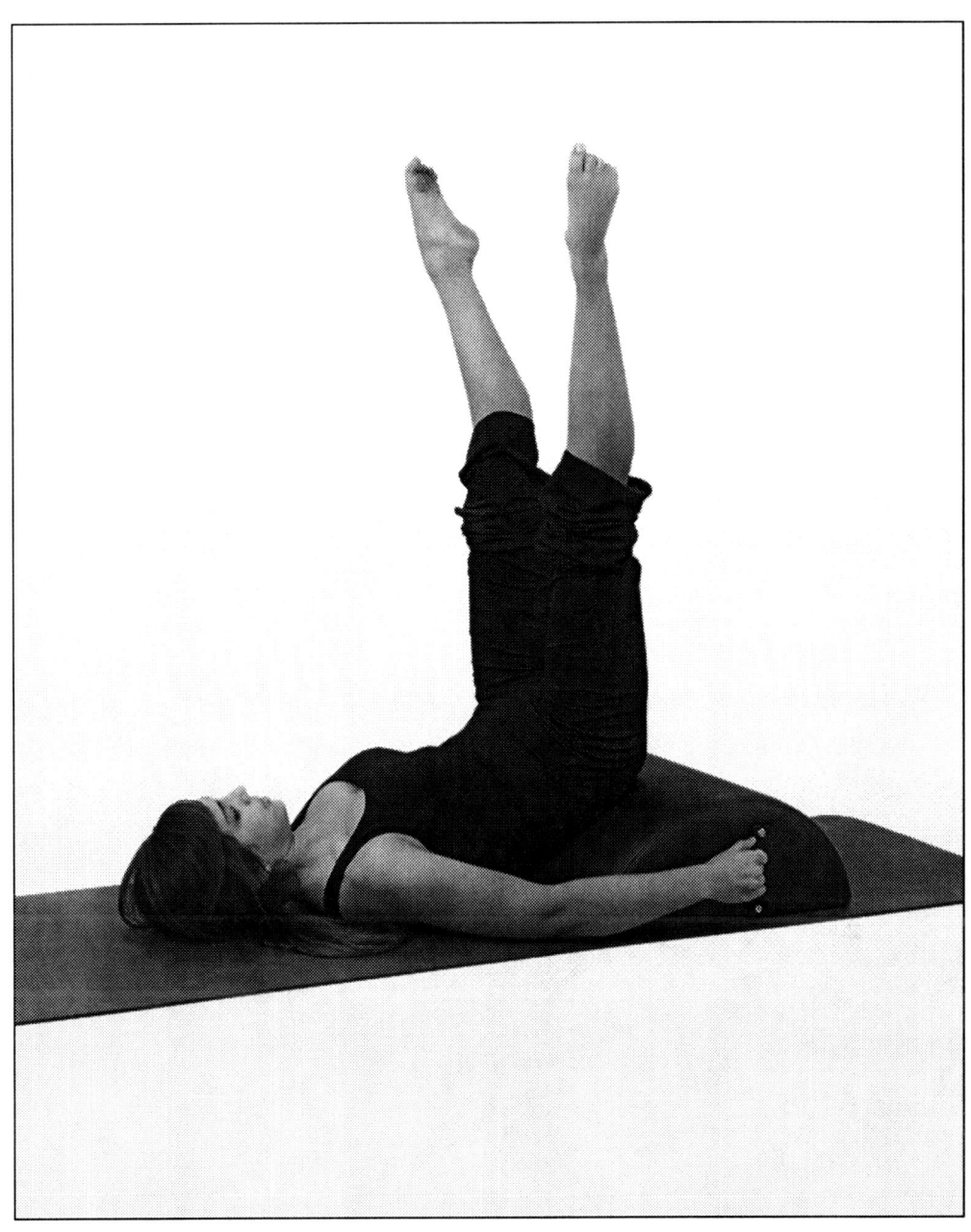

Scissors

Category: Hip mobility; disassociation of hip and spinal movement

Benefits: This exercise will improve the mobility of the hips and the control of the pelvis.

Set-Up: Lie supine with your buttocks against the barrel. Draw your knees to your chest as you pull the barrel under you to support your lower back. Hold the side handles as you lengthen your neck and extend your legs up in neutral.

Movement: While holding the handles and maintaining contact with the barrel for spine support, flex one hip as you extend the other. Attempt to keep your knees fully extended and your ribs in line with your ASIS. Hold this position for a few seconds while reaching long through your arches and then switch your leg position. Continue for the desired repetitions and then draw both knees to your chest to push the barrel away.

Cues:

- Reach long out of your legs.
- Relax your neck, and reach long out of the top back of your head.
- Keep the bottom of your sacrum against the barrel to maintain lumbar support.
- Keep sinking your navel to your spine.
- Do not allow your pelvis to slip into a posterior tilt.

Modification: Bend the knees slightly, and continue to move from the hip.

Breathing: Alternate your inhale and exhale as you switch the position of your legs like scissors

Repetitions: 5 to 8

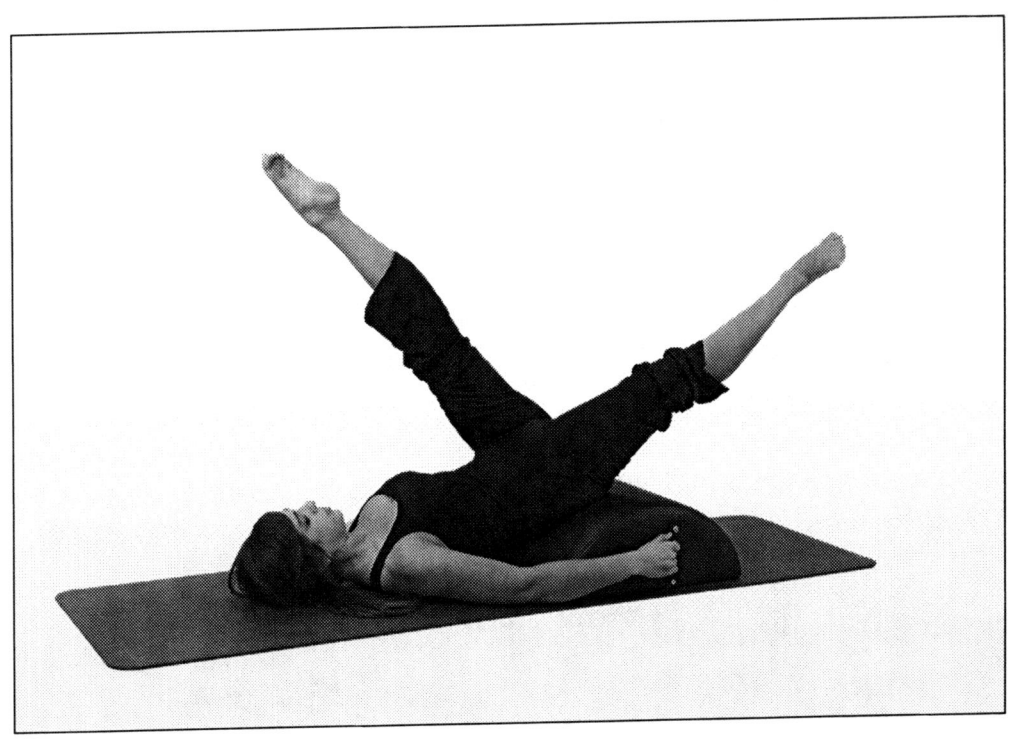

Walking

Category: Hip mobility; disassociation of hip and spinal movement

Benefits: This exercise will improve the mobility of the hips, control of the pelvis, and the stability of the core.

Set-Up: Lie supine with your buttocks against the barrel. Draw your knees to your chest as you pull the barrel under you to support your lower back. Hold the side handles as you lengthen your neck and extend your legs up in a neutral position.

Movement: While holding the handles and keeping contact with the barrel for spine support, alternate the legs in a small walking motion. Continue this motion as you walk from the ceiling down toward the mat and then back up to the ceiling. Repeat for the desired repetitions, and then draw the knees to the chest to push the barrel away.

Cues:

- Reach long out of your legs.
- Relax your neck and reach long out of the top back of your head.
- Keep the bottom of your sacrum against the barrel to maintain lumbar support.
- Keep your hips in neutral rotation.

Modification: Walk at just one position in the range of motion.

Breathing: Inhale and exhale smoothly as you perform the walking motion. On the exhale, reinforce the navel drawing into the barrel.

Repetitions: 5 to 8

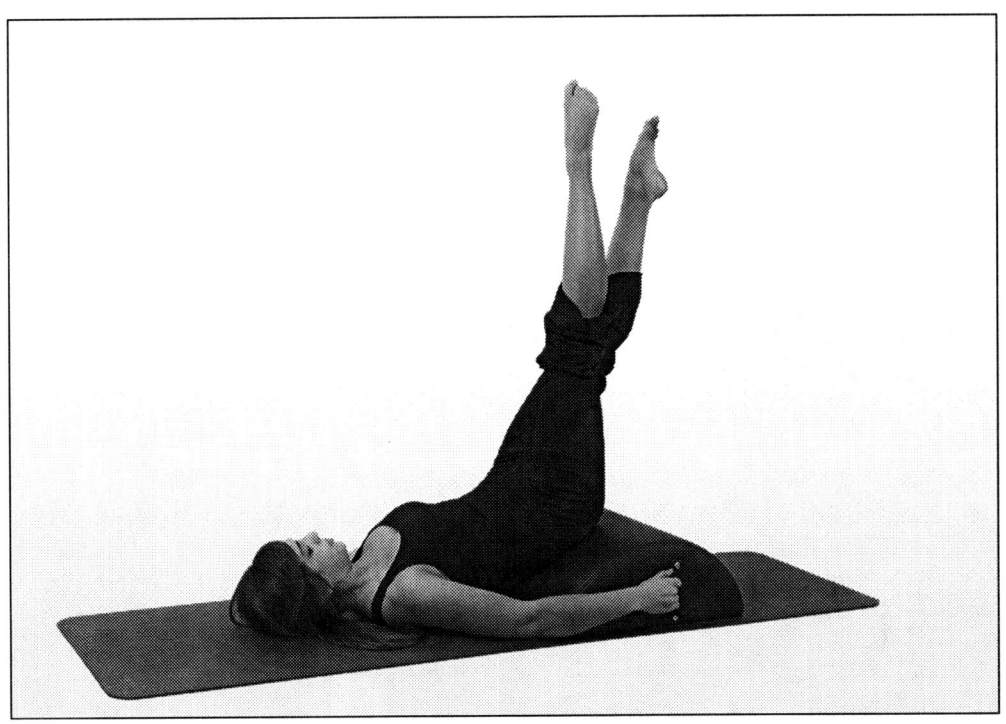

Bicycle

Category: Hip mobility; disassociation of hip and spinal movement

Benefits: This exercise will improve the mobility of the hips and the control of the pelvis. This exercise is especially useful for gently lengthening the hip flexors.

Set-Up: Lie supine with your buttocks against the barrel. Draw your knees to your chest as you pull the barrel under you to support your lower back. Hold the side handles as you lengthen your neck and extend one leg to the ceiling and one leg out above the floor. Position your hips in neutral rotation.

Movement: Begin by bending your knee of the lower leg and drawing your knee toward your chest while lowering the straight leg toward the mat. Continue to hold the handles and keep contact with the barrel for spine support. Repeat these motions to finish the cycle, and continue for the desired repetitions.

Cues:

- Reach long out of your legs.
- Relax your neck and reach long out of the top back of your head.
- Keep the bottom of your sacrum against the barrel to maintain lumbar support.
- Maintain knee-and-second-toe alignment.

Variation: Add interest by performing the exercise with flexed feet. To open the hip, hold the position when the lower leg is flexed at the knee.

Breathing: Inhale and exhale smoothly as you perform the cycling motion. On the exhale, reinforce your navel drawing into the barrel.

Repetitions: 5 to 8

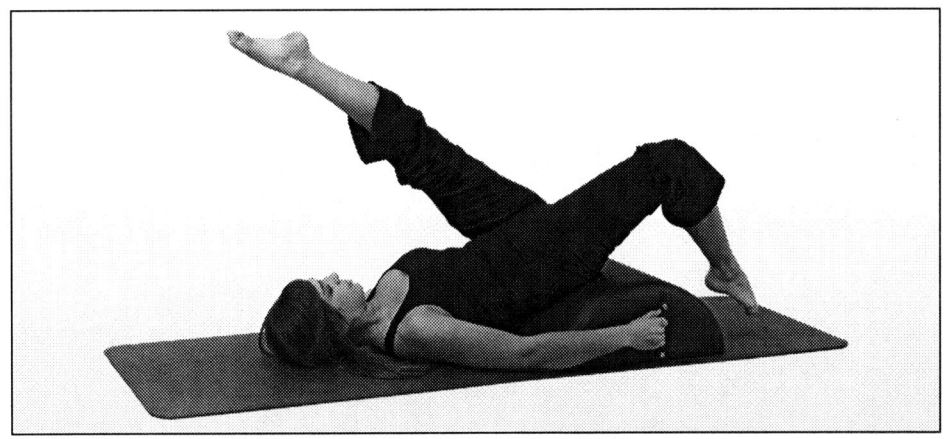

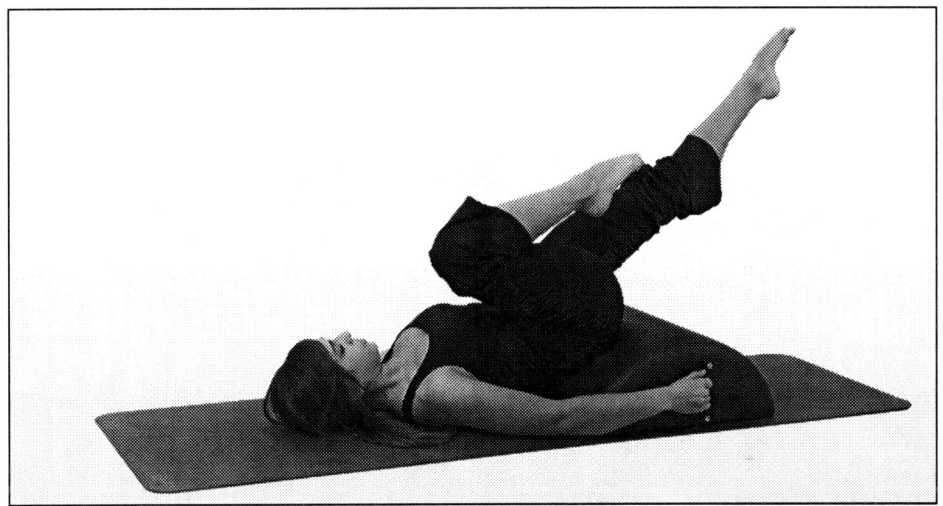

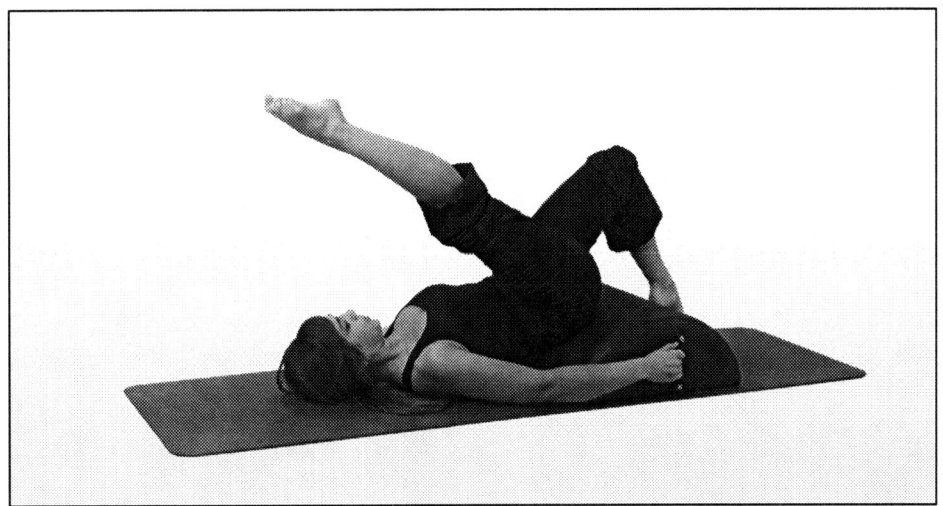

Beats

Category: Hip mobility; disassociation of hip and spinal movement

Benefits: This exercise will improve hip-adductor and pelvic-floor strength and control.

Set-Up: Lie supine with your buttocks against the barrel. Draw your knees to your chest as you pull the barrel under you to support your lower back. Hold the side handles as you lengthen your neck and extend your legs up in outward rotation.

Movement: While holding the handles and keeping contact with the barrel for spine support, abduct your legs and begin to beat your heels toward one another. Stop your heels from hitting one another at about 1 centimeter apart. The motion should be fast and powerful.

Cues:

- Reach long out of your legs.
- Relax your neck and reach long out of the top back of your head.
- Keep the bottom of your sacrum against the barrel to maintain lumbar support.
- Draw up and in with your inner thighs, and zip and wrap at the hips.

Variation: Perform this with either a flexed or pointed foot. Avoid sickling at the foot.

Breathing: Inhale and exhale smoothly as you perform the beats. Reinforce your navel to spine each time that you exhale.

Repetitions: 5 to 8

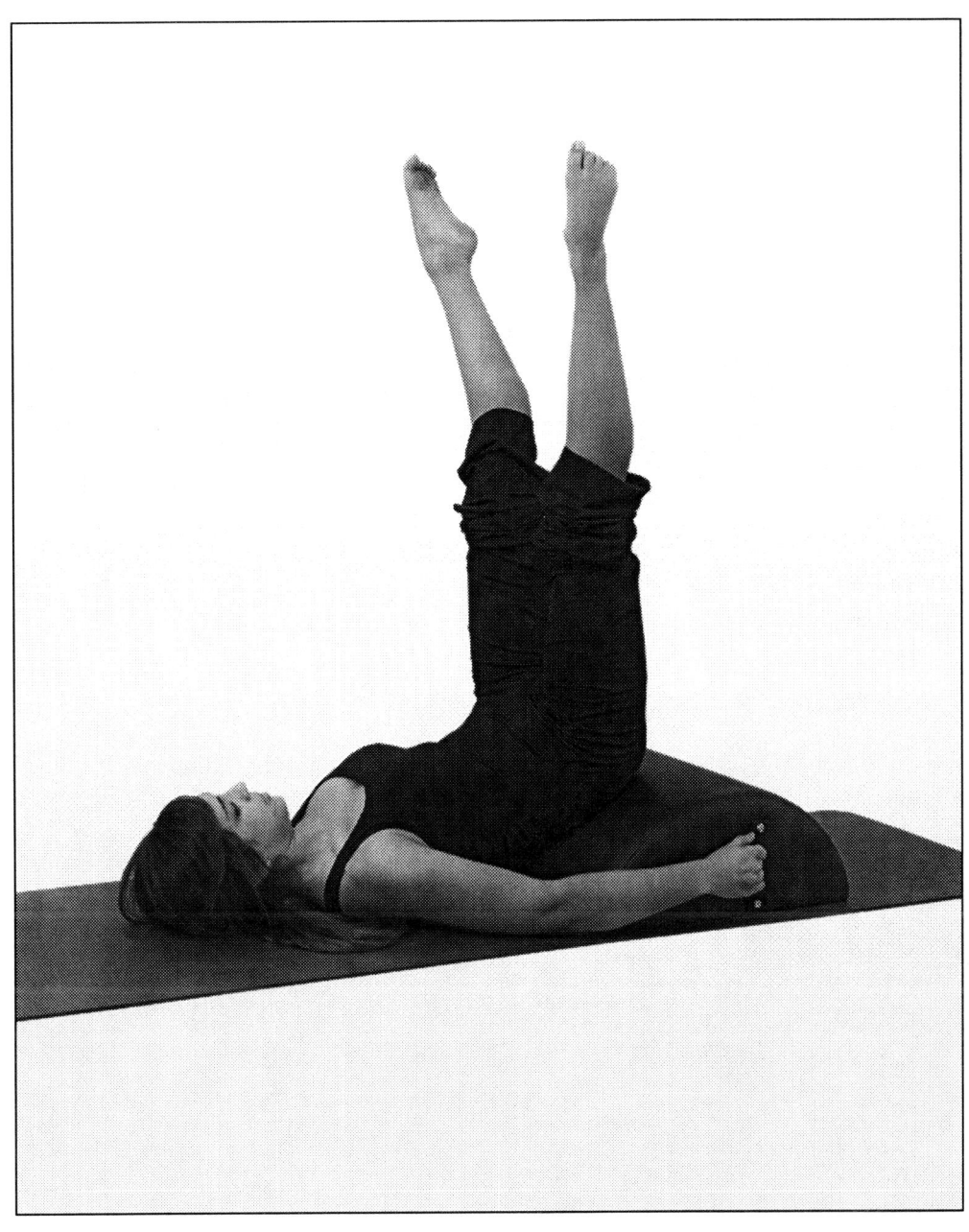

Rolling In and Out

Category: Lumbar mobility; disassociation of hip and spinal movement

Benefits: This exercise will improve the mobility of the lumbar spine and core stability.

Set-Up: Lie supine with your buttocks against the barrel. Draw your knees to your chest as you pull the barrel under you to support your lower back. Hold the side handles as you lengthen your neck.

Movement: While holding the handles and maintaining contact with the barrel for spine support, draw your knees toward your right ear. Then rock your knees toward your left ear. Repeat this motion for the desired repetitions and then draw your legs down to push the barrel away.

Cues:

- Keep the knees together.
- Relax your neck, and reach long out of the top back of your head.
- Keep the bottom of your sacrum against the barrel to maintain lumbar support. Your ribcage should be stable with no rotation.

Variation: Use a small ball between the knees to assist with the adduction of the legs and engage the pelvic-floor muscles.

Breathing: Inhale, as you bring your legs down and together. Exhale as you bring your legs to your right ear. Inhale to center, and exhale as you go toward your left ear.

Repetitions: 5 to 8

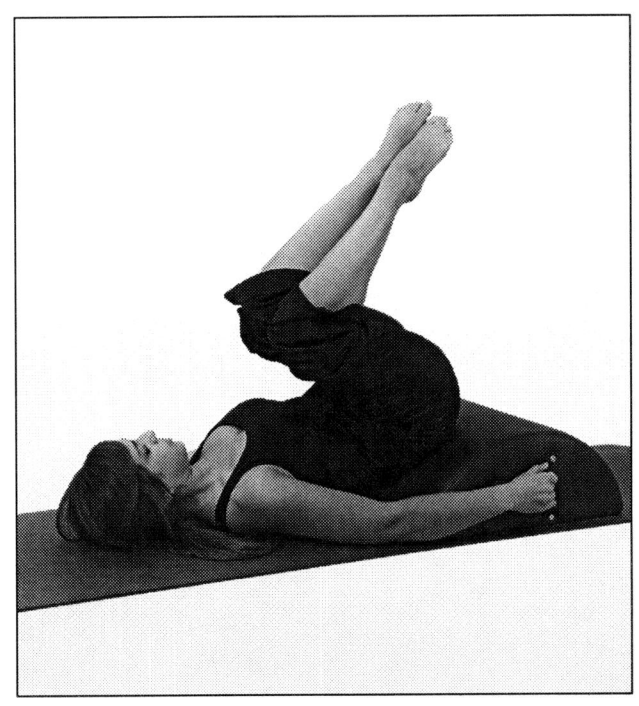
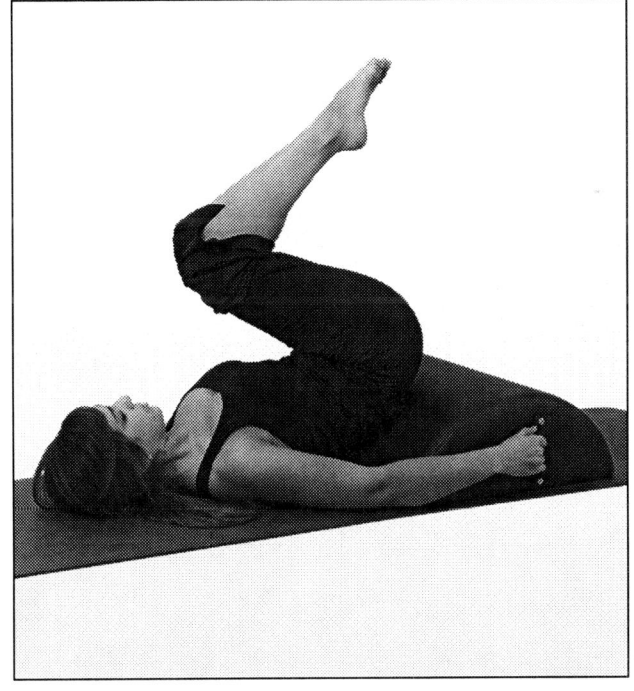

Appendix:
Adding Props to Your Pilates Mat Work

It is important to remember that props are an addition to your mat program. Creating an entire class using a prop for every exercise can become overwhelming for the teacher and the student. Many of the exercises using props are challenging and should be dispersed throughout a workout. The flow and variety of the Pilates class should continue with props as an addition only when needed for challenge or instruction. Avoid the temptation to disrupt the flow of the class with too many props in one class or to add so much challenge that the core muscles cannot engage properly. Instead, use the barrel, the ring, and the roller to enhance your present mat class one exercise at a time. Following are some sample class plans using the ring, the foam roller, the baby arc, and the spine corrector.

Workout #1
Articulating bridge (ring)
Cervical nod (ring)
Roll up (ring)
Hundred (ring)
Single-leg stretch
Double-leg stretch
Criss-cross
Leg circle
Scissors (roller)
Helicopter (roller)
Side plank
Side-lying up and down
Side-lying passé
Plank (roller)
Side plank
Side-lying up and down
Side-lying passé
Mermaid (roller)
Standing footwork (ring)

Workout #2
Articulating bridge (roller)
Ribcage arms (roller)
Hundred (roller)
Leg circle (roller)
Roll-up
Seated twist
Saw
Shave head (ring)
Rolling like a ball
Seal
Side-lying abduction (roller)
Side-lying adduction (roller)
Side plank on elbow
Modified swan dive
Single-leg kick
Side-lying abduction (roller)
Side-lying adduction (roller)
Side plank on elbow
Squats (ring)
Long back stretch (ring)
Footwork (ring)

Workout #3
Standing footwork (ring)
Articulating bridge (ring)
Cervical nod (ring)
Hundred (ring)
Arm circles (baby arc)
Leg circles (baby arc)
Scissors (baby arc)
Helicopter (baby arc)
Beats (baby arc)
Rolling in and out (baby arc)
Knee stretch (roller)
Cat (roller)
Push up (roller)
Roll up (spine corrector)
Teaser (spine corrector)
Swimming (spine corrector)
Mermaid legs (spine corrector)
Mermaid (spine corrector)

About the Author

Christine Romani-Ruby, MPT, ATC is a rarity in the Pilates world—an experienced Pilates professional with a strong background in physical therapy and fitness. Christine has been a licensed physical therapist for 17 years, and an associate professor at California University of Pennsylvania in the physical therapy and exercise science programs for six years. She is gold certified as a Pilates instructor through the Pilates Method Alliance. An international presenter, Christine is the owner of Phi Pilates, and co-owner of Phi Pilates Studio. She has authored four books and produced 13 videos on Pilates. Her most recent interests are in Pilates as a wellness practice, Pilates as therapeutic exercise in the physical therapy environment, and Pilates in the development of the adolescent dancer.

Christine holds a master of science degree in physical therapy from Slippery Rock University, a double bachelor of science in natural science and exercise science from Indiana University of Pennsylvania, and a certificate in athletic training from West Chester University. Currently, Christine is a doctoral candidate at Indiana University of Pennsylvania.